Dearest Cathy,

Strength and Courage
on your healing
journey!

Peace & Love

Enlightenment is Letting Go!

Healing from Trauma, Addiction, and Multiple Loss

Teresa Naseba Marsh

authorHOUSE®

AuthorHouse™
1663 Liberty Drive
Bloomington, IN 47403
www.authorhouse.com
Phone: 1-800-839-8640

First published by AuthorHouse 5/28/2010

ISBN: 978-1-4520-2893-4 (e)
ISBN: 978-1-4520-2892-7 (sc)
ISBN: 978-1-4520-2891-0 (hc)

Library of Congress Control Number: 2010907339

Printed in the United States of America
Bloomington, Indiana

This book is printed on acid-free paper.

Cover painted by artist Catherine Jaftha.
Author photo by David Marsh.

Contents

Acknowledgments

I thank the Creator and all my ancestors who walked with me during the writing of this book.

Thank you, David, my best friend and husband, for your unconditional love and support.

Thank you, my dear children, Shireen, Reon and Catherine, for embracing my teachings and for contributing to the world.

Ashley and Helen, my son- and daughter-in-law, thank you for coming into our lives.

Thank you, Maya and Jordan, my two grandchildren. This is my gift to you.

I thank my mother, father, and grandmother, now in the spirit world for all their love and teachings.

I thank all my sisters and my late brother for their love and support.

Thanks to my father-in-law who always believed in and encouraged me.

Thank you, Hannah, my healer, for always believing in me.

I thank all my clients, especially those who contributed to the writing of this book.

I thank all my spiritual teachers and healers who directed me over the years and those who encouraged me to follow the path.

And finally, thank you, all my dear friends, yogis, yoginis, and the editors and staff of AuthorHouse for your support and for cheering me on.

Introduction

It was that dark night of September 11 that I experienced an epiphany that shook me to my core. This book is a result of my revelations.

As I returned home from work after a long day of tears, fears, and disbelief, my youngest daughter, who was a journalism major, was glued to the television, unable to escape the horrific images of the attack on the twin towers replaying over and over in front of her. She greeted me with fear and terror in her eyes. "Have you seen? Have you seen?" I turned off the television and held her, and she cried. I asked her not to watch any more and explained that she was being traumatized and wounded as she was watching the replaying video.

I am an immigrant mother from Cape Town, South Africa. I have seen it all. I was born into violence. I have witnessed the South African police open fire on our children in South Africa. I come from the wars. I came to Canada with my three teenage children as a single mother to protect my children and to heal. Indeed, I received healing. I started my healing journey in the office of a young female psychiatrist, Dr. Hannah Wilansky, and worked with her for eight solid years, meeting once a week. As a psychotherapist and a gifted healer, I know the depth of hurt and pain. I have been a victim and a witness.

At the time of the attack on the twin towers, I worked as a manager for the Substance Abuse Program for African Canadian and Caribbean Youth (SAPACCY), as well as in my private psychotherapy practice. In my private practice, I mainly treated clients healing from abuse- related trauma and addiction. On September 11, my phone wouldn't stop ringing. My clients in deep exposure therapy at that point were experiencing meltdowns watching the news and viewing this entire trauma on live television.

That night, as I was sitting and praying, a realization emerged deep from within me that changed my life. I realized that the entire universe, its people—us—are facing darkness that is greater than ever before in history. It dawned on me that we are all suffering collectively at a global level from past and present traumas. I was convinced of this realization when I witnessed America throwing bombs and food to the people in Afghanistan. I realized that humanity had the power to destroy itself with nuclear weapons in minutes. We as a nation are traumatized on a daily basis. Every five minutes of every day, a woman is raped in my country. My clients share horrific stories with me on a daily basis. We respond to our own trauma by hurting others and ourselves as long as we live through our wounds and as long as we do not seek healing. This global abuse continues. Daily in the news we and our young children are confronted with the reality of teenage suicide; rape; incest; child molestation; child and adult abuse; violence against children, men, and women; wars; bombings; hunger; starvation; earthquakes; plane crashes; floods; plagues; and life-threatening diseases.

During my prayers that night I asked, " Who talks about daily healing, peace, love, truth, justice, reciprocity, virtue, compassion, and caring?" I then realized that as a wounded nation, we are waiting to experience a naked truth, healing from the core of the spirit. As I prayed, I saw my own healing journey moving by like a film before my eyes, from childhood to that day, from Africa to Canada.

Then the gift came. My ancestors spoke through my heart:

> *Write, Teresa. Write this book about healing with a language from your heart, in honest, gentle, kind words, with sincere healing not just for the healer but also for the healed. Should it be that we are all*

wounded, then we can all heal collectively. Healing can only take place as we connect, like our ancestors did in their healing circles. Speak in the language of your ancestors and allow this by the telling of stories. You have the ability to write a truth and create new patterns of healing and transformation. The main condition is that you have to be honest with your connection to your spiritual self, so speak your truth.

These words spoke loud and clear in my soul, and I realized that the fierce power of imagination is a gift from the Creator. I agreed, and the next day I started to write.

This book is about the audacity and courage of men and women who transcended from the depths of suffering, trauma, addiction, loss, life-threatening illness, and atrocities to clarity, awareness, hope, healing, freedom, peace, and enlightenment. For when we are enlightened, we understand that life is suffering, death is suffering, birth is suffering, illness is suffering; that suffering comes from our ignorance, and growth from the acceptance of that fact. Buddha taught us about the eight-fold path and said that if there is a cause for suffering, then there is also a diagnosis, and with a diagnosis we can implement a treatment. In embracing that treatment, nothing else can come but healing, transformation, and enlightenment. (*Buddha's Teachings*, 2005). The men and women in this book who so willingly and courageously volunteered to have their stories told, came from a place of knowing what it was like to feel alone in a world that had become so hostile, unsafe, unforgiving, and even cruel. Although the clients have consented to contribute to this book, I have changed their names and some other details to protect their confidentiality. On their healing journeys, as they began to be heard, validated, and supported, they reconnected with their truths and the highest parts of their beings, spirits, souls, true selves, higher selves, or whatever we want to call them. When we take that internal journey, guided and supported by an enlightened witness, there is no other place to go but deeper and deeper until a freedom, an inner peace, the innocence, our birthright, and our truth or the Self meets us.

We are all wounded and whole at the same time. We need to feel connected to others in order to love, understand, grow, give, receive, and heal. Hence my ancestors sat around that sacred fire in their healing circles with the knowledge that we are all connected to the hoop of life. On that hoop of life there is a place for everyone, enough for everyone, and healing for all. We need those circles. We need to connect at levels on which the spirit can be nourished and sustained. We are all created by the divine. We are spiritual beings, but we have moved so far away from it, afraid to speak it or name it, because we were made to fear that truth. As I looked at every wounded human being who came for healing, I saw that the struggles were about wanting to be closer to their higher selves. I realized that the fight within was not about good and evil but about a search to find a way to transform. A wise sage once said that we need garbage to make compost. If we have no compost, we have nothing to nourish the beautiful gardens within. We need the suffering and the affliction because they are organic, and therefore we can transform them. When we get hurt, we dislocate and disconnect, and we begin to identify with the wounds and pain. And if we continue to look away, the wounds become wounds that bleed no more, and we begin to hurt others and ourselves. In order to transcend all of the chaos and pain we need to be awake, conscious, and aware. Once that is achieved all the rest will fall into place.

This book is about that journey within. In this book, I discuss how, through the spoken word, honesty about our spiritual connection, poetry, and storytelling, we can seek at a deep level to heal the hurts, suffering, and pain. When we acknowledge past pain and suffering, we transform; this is the first step to healing. In step two we commit to the work that is required; in the stories that are included, you will witness the hard work and change that must occur for us to move from darkness to the light. Step three is about taking that honest and sincere journey within, each individual moving into the heart of the matter to find his or her true self.

On this journey we surrender; thus deep healing from the painful past wounds and suffering comes about. These gifts are hidden in the stories. The stories carry the gifts of deliverance; they are the stories of others who came before us or those who are with us, living among us. My hope is that the honesty, love, humanness, audacity, and courage of others will give each of us the courage to say, "Yes, we want to heal. We want this world to be a better place for our children, and our children's children." I believe in the healing power of love and will never cease to say that anything that is loved can be healed. Fellow human being, may you find what you were looking for when you picked up this book. May your soul and mind open up and embrace what you need to embrace. May you become a vessel of healing for another. Peace, joy, love, and blessings always.

Teresa Naseba Marsh

Chapter One

Trauma and Addiction

Introduction

This chapter offers a framework for the exploration of the complex connections between people with substance use disorders and trauma. Taking into account the distinct differences between the needs of men and women, with gender sensitivity, the chapter will cover the sequelae of trauma and addiction and unique innovative, integrative approaches to care.

Trauma and Addiction: The Connection

The relationship between trauma and substance use disorders has been well documented. Studies have found that 25 percent to 40 percent of patients receiving treatment for addiction report a history of trauma and present with clinically significant posttraumatic stress disorder (PTSD) symptomatology (Brief, Weathers, Krinsley, Young, and Kelly 1992; Brown and Wolfe 1994; Kovack 1986; Miller, Downs, and Testa 1993; Triffleman, Marmar, Delucci, and Ronfeldt 1995). Dual diagnosis of PTSD and a substance use disorder is surprisingly common. The rate of PTSD among patients in addiction treatment is 12 to 34 percent; for women it is 30 to 59 percent. Rates of lifetime trauma are even more common (Kessler, Sonnega, Bromet, Hughes, and Nelson 1995; Langeland and Hartgers 1998; Najavits, Weiss, and Shaw 1997; Steward 1996; Stewart, Conrod, Pihl, and Dongier 1999; Triffleman 1998).

Epidemiological studies in the United States have reported prevalence rates for substance abuse and dependence (including alcohol) of 20 percent in the general community. A systematic study reveals the high frequency of trauma history in addicted populations (Bernstein 1994; Boyd, Blow, and Orgain 1993; Cottler et al. 1990; Schnitt and Nocks 1984). Efforts are increasing to understand the complex relationships and devise effective interventions.

Other studies show that an individual with a past or current psychiatric disorder has a substantially increased risk for a substance use disorder. The risk is at least double for those with affective and anxiety disorders and is often higher for other psychiatric disorders.

Becoming abstinent from substances does not resolve PTSD; indeed, some PTSD symptoms become worse with abstinence (Brady, Killeen, Saladin, Dansky, and Becker 1994; Kofoed, Friedman, and Peck 1993; Root 1989).

People with PTSD and substance abuse or dependence are vulnerable to repeated traumas and more so than with substance use alone (Fullilove et al 1993; Herman 1992; Dansky, Byrne, and Brady 1999; Najavits et al 1998).

Perpetrators of violent assaults use substances at the time of assault in a high percentage of domestic abuse (50 percent) and rape (39 percent) cases (Bureau of Justice Statistics 1992).

Trauma Defined

People are traumatized either directly or indirectly, according to the DSM-1V diagnosis of PTSD. People can be traumatized without actually being physically harmed or threatened by harm. Simply learning about traumatic events carries traumatic potential.

What Is Posttraumatic Stress Disorder (PTSD)?

PTSD is the result of exposure to a traumatic or extremely emotionally and psychologically distressing event or events. Such an experience can have severe effects on a person's behavior, thinking, and feelings even long after the event or events have occurred. This can last for many years.

Many clients, as you will read in the following chapters,

believe or feel that the traumas were not that severe, and they really downplay them when they come for help. This denial of the seriousness of the events is part and parcel of the coping that comes into place during these events.

There Are Different Kinds of PTSD

Simple PTSD

This results from a one-time terrible event such as a rape or a car accident. This type is different from complex posttraumatic stress, which is described below.

Complex PTSD

This tends to occur when the abuse suffered was prolonged or repeated and/or if it was caused by a family member, loved one, or caregiver. It is also more prevalent if the abuse happened early in life. It can also happen as a result of chronic trauma or abuse in adult life, for example in a man or women involved in an abusive relationship for many years. In order to carry the diagnosis of PTSD, the following four things must be present:

    A. Experiencing an event that was life-threatening or that actually resulted in harm, intense fear, helplessness, or horror;

    B. Continuing to experience the traumatic event after it is over;

    C. Seeking to avoid reminders of the event; and

    D. Exhibiting signs of persistent arousal.

Sequelae of Trauma

Complex Posttraumatic Stress Response: DESNOS/Disorder of Extreme Stress, Not Otherwise Specified

Dr. Judith Herman and others state that severely traumatized individuals (for example, victims of severe childhood abuse, political torture, or concentration camps) have a more complex symptom picture (Herman 1992).

Responses to complex posttraumatic stress may include:

1. Affect dysregulation
   - Chronic preoccupation with suicide
   - Self-injury
   - Overreaction to minor stresses
   - Becoming emotionally and cognitively overwhelmed easily
   - Difficulty in calming or soothing self
   - Alcohol and other substance use
   - Problems with eating
   - Compulsive sexual activity
2. Dissociation and changes in consciousness
   - Amnesia
   - Transient dissociative episodes and depersonalization
   - Derealization
   - Reliving the experience
3. Changes in self-perception
   - Ineffectiveness
   - Guilt and responsibility
   - Shame
   - Helplessness
   - Self-blame
   - Feeling that nobody else understands
   - Minimizing the experience
4. Alterations in relations with others
   - Inability to trust
   - Revictimization
   - Victimizing others
   - Failures of self-protection
5. Somatization
   - Digestive system problems
   - Chronic pain
   - Cardiopulmonary symptoms
   - Conversion symptoms

- Sexual symptoms
6. Alterations in systems of meaning
   - Despair and hopelessness
   - Loss of previously sustaining beliefs
   - Loss of hope

Addiction Defined

Drug addiction is the chronic or habitual use of any chemical substance to alter states of body or mind for purposes that are not medically warranted.

Traditional definitions of addiction, with their criteria of physical dependence and withdrawal have been modified with increased understanding and research; with the introduction of new drugs, such as cocaine, that are psychologically or neuropsychologically addicting; and with the realization that its stereotypical application to opiate-drug users was invalid because many of them remain occasional users with no physical dependence.

Addiction is now more often defined by the continuing, compulsive nature of the drug use despite physical and/or psychological harm to the user and society and includes both licit and illicit drugs. The term "substance dependence" is now frequently used because of the broad range of substances (including alcohol and inhalants) that can fit the addictive profile.

Psychological dependence is the subjective feeling that the user needs the drug to maintain a feeling of well-being. Physical dependence is characterized by tolerance (the need for increasingly larger doses in order to achieve the initial effect) and withdrawal symptoms when the user is abstinent.

The United States has the highest substance use rate of any industrialized nation. Government statistics show that 47 percent of the United States population has tried marijuana, cocaine, or some other illicit drug. By comparison, 65 percent of the population has smoked cigarettes, and 82 percent have tried alcoholic beverages. Marijuana is the most commonly used illicit drug (Substance Abuse and Mental Health Services Administration 2009).

Why Do People Use Drugs?

People take drugs for many reasons: peer pressure, stress relief, increased energy, relaxation, pain relief, escape from reality, greater feelings of self-esteem, and recreation. They may take stimulants to keep alert or cocaine for the feeling of excitement it produces.

Effects of Substance Use

The effects of substance use can be felt on many levels: on the individual, on friends and family, and on society. People who use drugs experience a wide array of physical effects other than those expected. The excitement of a cocaine high, for instance, is followed by a "crash": a period of anxiety, fatigue, depression, and an acute desire for more cocaine to alleviate the feelings of the crash. Cannabis and alcohol interfere with motor control and are factors in many automobile accidents. Users of marijuana and hallucinogenic drugs may experience flashbacks, unwanted recurrences of the drug's effects weeks or months after use. Sudden abstinence from certain drugs results in withdrawal symptoms. Heroin withdrawal can cause vomiting, muscle cramps, convulsions, and anxiety. With the continued use of a physically addictive drug, tolerance develops, that is, constantly increasing amounts of the drug are needed to duplicate the initial effect.

Sharing hypodermic needles used to inject some drugs dramatically increases the risk of contracting HIV infection and viral hepatitis. In addition, both prostitution and the disinhibiting effect of some drugs put users at higher risk of acquiring HIV and other sexually transmitted diseases. Because the purity and dosage of illegal drugs are uncontrolled, drug overdose is a constant risk. There are over ten thousand deaths directly attributable to drug use in the United States every year; the substances most frequently involved are cocaine, heroin, and morphine, often combined with alcohol, tobacco, or other drugs. Many drug users engage in criminal activity, such as burglary and prostitution, to raise the money to buy drugs; and some drugs, especially alcohol, are associated with violent behavior.

Treatment

The Therapeutic Alliance or Relationship

This is the most crucial aspect in therapy; it is the positive connection that must be established before anything else can happen. This relationship is the key that will open the door to the work that has to be done. The healing lies within that therapeutic relationship. The issues of safety and trust must be considered at all times. People bring with them their suffering, hurt, pain, guilt, shame, helplessness, hopelessness; and in these symptoms they tell us how bad it was and still is. A compassionate, caring, and giving professional with deep knowledge and skills can support and assist people on their healing journey.

Stages of Addiction Treatment

Stage One: Engagement, Stabilization, Detoxification, and Contracting

All of the above entail the building of trust in the relationship, coupled with empathy, understanding and respect. Looking at issues such as housing, transportation, and welfare, the involvement of significant others is key to the healing journey. Psychoeducational sessions are crucial as we educate and talk about the substances and effects on the person's life. Reflective listening and the exploration of the fears of quitting are mandatory in this first phase of treatment.

Stage Two: Persuasion, Empathy, Support, and Psychoeducation

Here we focus on motivational interviewing, acknowledgement of the struggles and pain, and exploration of the benefits of quitting. The therapist's understanding and empathy at this stage is crucial. Education follows all the stages and moves through the treatment of both trauma and addiction as a golden thread. The education must focus on all the dimensions of the human being: mind, body, and spirit. We also explore the need for pharmacotherapy at this stage and implement that as soon as possible.

Stage Three: Active Treatment

In this stage we focus on all the skills and interventions that could help and enhance recovery. Clients may need to go into residential treatment or attend AA, NA, or other therapy groups that focus on addiction and trauma. Pharmacological support remains an important part of the treatment. The teaching of new skills to deal with all the challenges cannot be emphasized enough.

Stage Four

Here we solidify all the gains of the previous stages through continual exposure to the triggers and challenges that come on a day-to-day basis. Addiction treatment is a process, as is trauma treatment. We walk with people all the way and collaboratively figure out what is working for them. Each and every individual will present with their own particulars and idiosyncrasies and working hand in hand with people can empower them to become stronger and more motivated.

In chapter thirteen, which covers group psychotherapy for trauma and addiction, the interventions and treatment strategies useful in dealing with both disorders are discussed in more detail.

Stages of Trauma Treatment

Stage One (Early Stage): Stabilizing and Managing Trauma

SAFER

S: Safety and Self-Care. The first step to any form of trauma treatment is safety and self-care. Here we teach clients to manage the symptoms and to gain the knowledge to be empowered or to get stronger in the process. Safety includes ensuring safe housing and checking and talking about suicidal ideation. It is also important to schedule a physical examination and make sure that no signs or symptoms are missed. This also includes the use and implementation of pharmacotherapy.

A: Affect. Many clients are stunned when they hear for the first time that all their symptoms and behaviors have names. When they grasp this and realize that they are not crazy or imagining things, they begin to heal. Those symptoms persist, as I explain in many of the chapters, as a language, that is, being able to speak about the unspeakable.

F: Function. This is about recognizing the old ways of hurting self, by self-harm or by using drugs and alcohol and then moving toward making changes to function at a higher level of being.

E: Education. This tool is woven through both trauma and addiction like a golden thread. When clients begin to understand the why of their feelings, thoughts, and behaviors, they can begin to make informed decisions to change.

R: Relationships. In all the chapters on trauma and addiction, the areas of relationships are discussed in detail. Life is about relationships: the relationships with self, partners, family, friends, and the world. Both disorders involve and affect all of the above, hence my inspiration to write this book after the brutal experience of 9/11.

Stage Two (Middle Stage): Processing and Grieving Traumatic Memories

During this stage the exploration of the past and painful memories is initiated. We explore how the trauma affected the past and also how it affects the individual in the here and now.

Various approaches may be used in this stage, including exposure, cognitive process therapy, desensitization, and eye movement desensitization reprocessing (EMDR). I have written in many of the chapters about the importance of alternative therapies such as yoga, meditation, thought tracking, and group therapy. (There are more explanations in chapter thirteen, which discusses group psychotherapy for trauma and addiction).

Stage Three: Restructuring, Reconnecting, Rebuilding, and Reintegrating

During this stage the focus is on the above-mentioned four Rs. This is the ongoing work, and the goal here is to encourage people to let go. Letting go of all dysfunctional ways in order to build new healthy lives and ways of living. This stage is beautifully written about by people in this book who took the risk of telling their stories. Giving back to humanity and society as they did is a clear indication of the extent of their healing and transformation.

Conclusion

As we move into the new era of multiple technological advancements, we continue to encounter the vulnerability and suffering of humans whose childhood abuse histories led to the development of complex posttraumatic stress disorder and addiction. These disorders brings with them challenging, complicated, and painful consequences. These challenges must be addressed at all levels—mind, body, and spirit—in other words, in the context of the biological, psychological, spiritual, and social dimensions.

Treatment should be client-centered, gender-sensitive, and specific to the needs of people being aware of the complexity of needs. Treatment must be integrative, inclusive, diverse, effective, collaborative, and consistent with new research and best practices.

Health care professionals are challenged daily working in this field and need sound knowledge, skills, and gentle openness, coupled with deep compassion and understanding of the human spirit and suffering. Self-care is mandatory for the professional in this field. The healing and deep work only happen in the therapeutic relationship. Professionals should treat themselves in the same way they advocate for their clients, maintaining safety, self-care, and deep compassion. Anything that is loved can be healed.

Chapter Two

My Story

Introduction

I was born in South Africa to parents who were both very strong and faithful followers of Islam. Although my ancestors were slaves, my father supported his wife and nine children with the income from his own business, selling fruit, fish, and vegetables. I was the seventh child in a close-knit family, a group of eight girls and one boy. I had two step-siblings from my mom's first relationship, but they lived with their grandmother. We as a family experienced the pain and suffering of living under the apartheid regime. We were all exposed to the Group Areas Act, brutal racism, numerous riots, and the violent deaths of friends and close family members.

With this background, I had no choice but to grow up fast, and at the age of seventeen, I started my nursing career. My dream at that time was to unite all people, irrespective of race, color, or creed, to nurse people as human beings and not according to color codes. I was fortunate enough to see my dreams largely realized, as I was one of the first black nurses to care for white patients in South Africa. Later, I became one of the first black instructors of white and nonwhite nursing students at Groote Schuur Hospital, the leading hospital in the country where Professor Christiaan Barnard performed the first heart transplant.

The first ten years of my career challenged me as a wife, mother, and career woman. During my five years of training—three years of basic nursing and one year each of post-basic training in midwifery and psychiatry—I converted to Christianity, married, and had three children. Then only twenty-three years old, I became a senior nurse. I remember my time in psychiatry, working in a crisis unit attached to an emergency unit, carrying a caseload of patients in time-limited, crisis intervention. At the time I supervised student psychiatrist nurses, medical students, and psychiatrists in residency. It was a challenging task confronting the effects of drug and alcohol addiction, interracial violence, and institutional racism on the lives of individuals and families.

1979 brought many changes in my personal and professional life. My marriage ended during that year, and I became the sole supporter of my three children, then ages three, seven, and eight. It was during this time that the head of post-basic nursing education asked me to initiate an oncology program for registered nurses. Years later I also began studying toward my undergraduate degree in nursing education and community health nursing science at the University of South Africa.

In the next twelve years I embraced hard work in curriculum design, planning, and implementation. I designed and taught a year-long, full-time course in oncology nursing that attracted students from throughout South Africa, neighboring countries, and as far away as Taiwan. Oncology nursing also opened international doors for me. I became a speaker at national and international conferences in England, Europe, and North America. The government of Lesotho invited me to establish a national program of detection, screening, and prevention of cervical cancer in that country. Shortly after Namibia gained independence, I helped run oncology workshops there for exiled health care workers returning to their war-torn country. I also, with one of my students, coauthored the first oncology textbook for health care professionals in South Africa.

I left South Africa in 1992, as a single mother with three children ages fifteen, nineteen, and twenty. The prime motivation in my decision to leave was my desire to offer my children the opportunity for education and freedom. Despite my accomplishments, the democratization of the political process, and the advances in abolishing apartheid, I experienced poverty in my life in totality:

physically, emotionally, spiritually, culturally, and socially. It was only after moving to Canada that I experienced true freedom, away from the censors, away from state-controlled media, away from the watchful eyes of the South African police, away from the injustice of gross economic inequality, and away from brutal violence.

My first three years in Toronto were very busy. Initially I worked as an oncology nurse at Mount Sinai Hospital and taught part-time in the Faculty of Continuing Education at Centennial College. I married a Canadian physician who specialized in addiction and psychotherapy. My husband, David, and I had the privilege of being co-therapists for a group therapy process for patients suffering from multiple losses.

My early years in Canada also offered me educational opportunities I never had in South Africa. As I moved my career back to psychiatric nursing, I embarked upon a master's degree in psychology through the Adler School of Professional Psychology.

Moving Into More Personal Details

I don't know how many people move into doing this work because of their own experiences and journeys. I know that I had no choice; I was chosen. My mother told me this story many times: I was born premature at seven months and was so tiny I had to be nursed in a shoebox, covered with cotton wool for the first two months of my life. She said that her midwife, Nurse Kakana, who had delivered all my siblings, told her when I was born, "Asa, here is my nurse, my healer, my prem. She finally arrived." Whenever my mother told me this story, I would always ask her how Nurse Kakana knew that I was the one. Mother said that she did not know but remembered so clearly the joy on her midwife's face, knowing that I was the one to carry on her work. From there on, Mom said, all I could talk about from a very young age was to become a nurse.

"You took newspaper and made yourself an apron and a cap and pretended to be a nurse," Mom said. That is how it was for me from that time on. I was going to help people and take good care of them. And I did.

There was always this deep knowing that I had to help take away hurt and pain and love people. I remember my first day at school. I felt so big and so smart. Most of the kids cried when their parents left, and I wondered what was wrong with them. My teacher, Miss Abdullah, who became my teacher for the first three years of my life, was my inspiration, and I just simply adored her.

One day she took a good look at me. "Come here," she said. "You're going to help me lead these babies to the toilet." And there I was, in front of the line, walking the class to the toilet. I became the caretaker at age six. Miss Abdullah also told me that I was very smart, and indeed, during all my years of school, I was first in my classes. I was very proud.

I had a very happy childhood all in all. My father had his own business and sold fish and vegetables. He was always home for breakfast, lunch, and dinner. My mother was always home. I observed a great love between them and remember that every Friday he would present my mother with a bouquet of flowers. I could see the love in their eyes. They also had their fights, and sometimes my mother would leave for days. I remember I was so scared during those times because I did not know if she would come back. I also felt the pain of my dad and his unhappiness. She always came back, though, and we would all be happy again. I enjoyed all my siblings, and we had lots of fun together. There was the usual sibling rivalry of course, but all in all, my memories of that time are happy.

Then one day all that changed for me. I was nine years old. A family member molested me. It left me devastated and fearful, but I never told anyone. I feared my perpetrator, and I feared for my life. He told me he would kill me should I tell.

Many years later, when I was inspired by poetry writing and the spoken word, I wrote about it for the first time. After that I was inspired to write more as I began my own healing journey in Canada. These are excerpts from that first poem.

He Stole My Innocence

Mamma says, come you are going to be late
Look at your face; your hair is in an unmanageable state
Get dressed, put on your clothes, there ...
In my beautiful white dress, I still feel bare

Today in school, we celebrate the birth of the Prophet
We wear our best; we are all in white so pure
They serve special food and lots of sweets
The children get so excited when they see all the eats

Today I walked to school in my beautiful white dress
I am so dirty, touched, used inside I am a mess
Inside, outside all over me you see
Is his hands, breath, smell, I am no longer free

My dear teacher says, girl, "Where is the smile today?"
Inside my head a voice shouts, "Tell her, see what she says"
Maybe it is just some thing that happens to all
"Don't tell her, you dirty girl', another voice calls

I lay my head down on my desk, I am not well
She walks toward me, I think she can smell
That day as the celebrations continued on
My head, my heart, my feelings, my smile all gone

One thing I kept saying over and over again
He will never touch me again; I will remove his stain
But one thing I said to myself all the way
He will never touch me again, and I began to pray

I began to imagine that I told my mamma dear
It really helped me so, it took away the fear
In the middle of the night when the dreams came
I prayed again and again I prayed all the same

Comments

I had no idea at all how this affected me at the time, but I know I changed at a very deep level. I had terrible nightmares and sometimes sleepless nights. Since the perpetrator was a family member, I would freeze whenever he was around. I became very conscious of my body and my bum. I have "booty," like many black girls. I became ashamed of it and always tried to cover it up. It was difficult because the more I tried, the harder it became. Then the kids at school gave me the nickname *busman holle* (bushman bum), and that did it for me. It was a struggle for me until we came to Canada where everybody appreciated a nice booty. I was healed from that one!

The molestation was only a small part of the violence and abuse I witnessed and experienced. Growing up in South Africa was about witnessing violence on a daily basis. People almost began to view it as the norm.

The goal of this book is not to go on and on about the atrocities but rather to acknowledge their impact and their existence and then discuss how people heal from such trauma. This book is about how healing can come about.

As I said, my healing journey started in Toronto in the office of Hannah Wilansky, a female psychiatrist. She saved my life. She encouraged me by precept and example to become a psychotherapist. I was working at Mount Sinai at that time as an RN. I had already met David, and by then we were married. I became clinically depressed with suicidal ideation. I felt so guilty. There I was in beautiful Canada; the children were doing great; I was married to the most amazing man; but I was *so damn sad*. Why?

Well, the next poem will let you into the why.

They Love Me, They Understand Me

The first person I told about that man finally came
Thirty years later, a long time I lived with the shame
They say when you are unconditionally loved
You begin to heal from below and above

I can say to you those true words have proved
After I told my dearly beloved, I was so moved
See the perpetrator came to visit me in a dream again
I screamed in terror, I could feel the pain

Then a gentle voice told me it was only a dream
It was then that I stopped to scream
I looked up at him eyes full of tears
I uttered "he haunted me now for over 30 years"

My beautiful gentle man rocked me in his arms
I could hear distant drums, angels singing psalms
He said "tell me sweet heart, only if you want"
His compassion, understanding, caring and love, I was stunned

I slowly told my story through pain and tears
As I continued I felt less pain and fear
He continued to rock me back and forth
He whispered, "I love you, you are so much worth
He said, sweet heart you are safe with me
I am holding you now and I heard your plea

Now all the healing will come for you
Speak to your therapist, tell her your truth
I am here, she is there, and we care about you
At your side in spirit I am true

It grieves me to hear that you suffered so long
You are good woman, a good mother so strong
I admire your beauty, your passion your wit
You faced so much in your life, yet you never quit

The next day I tell my therapist how
The truth was finally out, that I wanted healing now!
I wept again and again as I re-experienced the pain
I feel so weak, my legs so lame

I bow my head in shame; I say, "It is so tough"
I have been depressed for a while now, how rough
I want to understand now why I suffered so
Since he took my innocence, the dramas just increased you know

She says in a gentle soft voice how brave was I
I say yes … but what about those times that I wanted to die?
But you did not; you protected yourself instead all the way
Listen my dear; listen to what I have to say

It was never your fault, you did nothing wrong
Your husband is right, you are so strong
With me here you are safe and can tell your entire story
Oh! This moment, right here right now I feel God's glory

I look in her soft eyes and I smile again
Since I am on my journey with this lady, I feel so sane
She understands me, she gets what I say
She gives me hope, every time for that new sunray

As I said when we are loved unconditionally so
We as human beings begin to grow and grow and grow
Until we can love ourselves and others into freedom
In peace then, we thus enter God's kingdom

Comments

I worked with Hannah for eight years. We met once a week in her office in Toronto. She witnessed my healing journey and accompanied me through all the challenges, personal, professional, and spiritual. As you can see, when we embark upon our healing journeys, life goes on. You continue to work, study, love, laugh, and live with a deeper joy and a determination so powerful. As you begin to understand yourself at such deep levels and the crusts that you build around the heart begin to soften and dissipate, you find your true self, or as I always say, you begin to realize that truth is your identity. I learned so much about myself in those healing sessions. I had no idea that a human being could repress so much pain and hurt.

I was also surprised to realize that my psyche was so in tune with what I was doing to heal. Most days I had to rush from one place to the next to be on time for my sessions. Then the minute I sat down and looked into the eyes of my healer, the tears would just come. Afterward I would venture with her toward more pain and more hurt that I was not even aware of. She would just sit there and listen with her heart. Indeed she was listening with the deepest part of her being. When it was time for her to console or to support me, she was always right on. I felt her love and care so often. I sensed her holding me as I peeled off layer after layer. Each time a layer was removed, I felt lighter; I had more clarity; I could often feel those hurts and pains leaving my body.

I was inspired to write this last poem soon after we moved to Vancouver. In this poem I truly connected with my inner child. It was profound and a rebirth.

Come Here, and Let Me Love You Forever

My inner child comes to life!
Look at you laughing, smiling, jumping and dancing on the earth
Your mouth so wide with love and joy, singing for this new birth
Yes the day has finally come for you my sweetness
Just feel, enjoy, experience and play in this beautiful bliss

Dance, sing, shout, roll, play and have fun
Our days of laughter, freedom and play have begun
Yes, too long it has been my dearest child
Look at you that grin that happiness, so wild
Come here let me kiss you and hold you forever near
We did it together, united we faced all the fear

Let me hold you and look at you again and again
Yes, I see the beautiful white dress is now with out a stain
Thank you for your gift of spirit and hope
From this day forth for whatever to come we will cope

I did not mean to hurt you or hide you so deep
Just wanted to make sure that you were safe to keep
The pain was so severe; I did not know better my dear
Now what is that look for … come over here

Let me love you and hold you again and again
Let me sing with you, shout with you, run in the rain
Oh remember the times we ran bare feet and all
Dad gave us fruit and melon, we ignored the dinner call

Those were the beautiful moments even in trouble with mom
Remember the time she screamed at us and took all our bubble gum
We just experienced the freedom, life and joy, life was so sweet and
great
Until that dark night, that cursed night when I entered that dark
state

All I knew then is that I had to protect that little girl
I knew that what she had was special, a shining pearl
Then one day I looked and I could not find you no more
I was devastated, my heart torn, the ache for years I walked with this
sore

Sometimes you came out and you just wanted to play a bit
Other days you just wept and wept, grieved in that dark pit
Girl the confusion drove me nuts some days, but I never gave up
Because all the time I sensed that we were drinking from the same
cup

This is the greatest gift that I received today
We are together, free forever, yet still I pray
Lord, please protect us, stay with us in this pure unity
Please confirm with us that this is reality

After all this time now united with you little girl
Look at you my beautiful shining pearl
Look at your face, your energy, and your glow
That's right, dance sing, shout let's put on that show

I know, I felt your presence when I danced and sang
In fear and protection I often closed the door with a bang
It must have hurt, it must have been hell, and I feel so sad
All right sweetness, I know now I have to rejoice and be glad

We are going to make up for all these lost years
The jubilee, the joy and happiness brings me to tears
From now on yes there will be many laughs and tears of bliss
So what do we call each other … I see sis and sis

Naseba, Teresa, Tanaka, Meisie, all the same
United joined together by love, courage and name
Many times I asked Abba "Why? Why? Why?"
When I saw you at first I was so shy

Then, on meeting I realized that Abba knew best
Thank you Abba, from this day forth we will do the rest
Our story will heal and rescue many a soul and heart
Let's continue to celebrate, meditate, this is the best start

When people see that we never gave up hope
They will embrace their pain and find healthy ways to cope
Oh sis, how I wish for a day of jubilee for all humanity
Mothers, fathers, sisters, brothers, community all in unity

That is my prayer, my dream Abba, so hear my call above
Compassion, Peace, trust, reciprocity, harmony above all LOVE
It was really love for each other that kept that flame burning
Trauma, hurt, pain, suffering and mistakes are all parts of learning
There are no mistakes in life, only lessons
With faith, trust and hope we all find our true essence

Conclusion

I struggled long and hard about writing my story. I prayed many times about it. Then one night I had dream. In that dream I realized that I was dreaming. All I could feel and see was transparent. In the work that I do, I am transparent. I then had the answer. This is a small portion of my life, my story. I believe in love and the healing power of love. I know that we cannot heal on our own. It is only when we receive the gift of true love that we begin to heal. I healed deeply because I believe in love. Thank you, Creator, David, my children, ancestors, parents, siblings, Hannah, universe, friends, clients, and world for your unending love.

Chapter Three

Addiction And Abuse

Introduction

The day after that revelation on the night of 9/11, I saw my first client in my private practice. I had been engaging in exposure trauma work with Christine. Christine was a twenty-seven-year-old black woman who had been born and raised in Canada. Her parents had immigrated to Canada from the Caribbean during the sixties. When she connected with me, she was heavily addicted to cannabis and problem drinking. She was unemployed, deeply depressed, and suicidal. She was seeking help for her abuse-related trauma and addiction. She was abused at a very young age by several perpetrators, and she had some memories related to her father's abuse. When she was older, she always ended up in abusive relationships.

On that visit she was extremely disturbed as she had flashbacks about her father abusing her. As she told her story, she became physically sick and nauseous in the office. As she remembered, more memories emerged. When she left the office, I sat in the room, still present with her hurt and laments.

My first poem below evolved from that moment, formed from the gentle language of my ancestors. I only put my pen down when I felt a sense of completion. The words just poured forth from my soul. I realized that I was writing first about the client and continued to respond in a second poem as her therapist. I was inspired with the poem titles in the same way as the words came forth. I accepted the inspiration as it came to me.

Missing Father
(The client speaks.)

Just today I realized that my father was never there
Only one birthday party of mine he attended, is that fair?
I suddenly remember a Cuddle and stroke
So revolting, so wrong. I just want to choke

Why are all these memories coming to me this day?
It is so painful, so confusing, will it forever stay?
He used me, abused me, and hurt me so much
Yet my body surrendered to his touch

Feelings and memories force me to contemplate
I loathe as I looked towards the open gate
He beat, teased me and manipulated me
I hated him, Mama. Why couldn't you see?

The absent father, he was never there
His visits, his presence in our lives so bare
Why is it that I see so clearly today?
Is it because I now often pray?

I want you to know exactly how I feel
Maybe you will think, what is the big deal?
My daddy gave me no love or hope
With his rejection I could not cope

I now see him beating and taunting me
Sometimes I cried and begged him to let me be
"Mother, he abused me, you never looked"
You were passive, or kept busy or cooked

I hated that man for the longest of time
I saw how he left Mama without a dime
When I told you Mama you said… "child I know"
So, if you knew, why did you not show?

By the time I was nine, he left us alone
My joy was so great I carved a message in stone
He was gone; he would never hurt me again
I looked up to the sky and it started to rain
I praised God; I thanked my Creator so loud
Mama was so sad, but I needed to shout

You Are Doing the Work
(The therapist speaks.)

As I listened to you today, sister dear
I know that your healing is so near
Two years ago when we met for the first time
You unemployed, lost and without a dime

You were scared, confused and so full of shame
Your wounds raw, you could not say your name
You explored your current life your state
You told me about your pain and self-hate

Through the weeks, months you persevered
You worked, looked, explored and questioned
Your pain was so deep, your wounds so raw
You showed me the hurt and opened the door

Today you ask these clear questions
All the answers you received and now
It is clear because you took the journey dear
With your eyes on the open wounds so clear

I am sorry that your father was never there
Your pain, anger, loss and hurt I share
Sometimes it's hard to understand the why
Therefore you suffered and wanted to die

As I said, it was never your fault
Yes the memories like rubbing salt
To the open wound already bleeding
I recall the times when you were pleading

Painful it was when Mama turned away
These new revelations are here to stay
In the two years you have worked so hard
You are healing, you are so smart

Today I can see that you are doing so well
You are healing, you are in the light, I can tell
Your courage will sustain you always
What an honor to give you praise

Comments

It dawned on me that, through poetry, I had embarked upon a new and profound way to support the healing journey of my clients. This was indeed a deeper spiritual way to teach, support, validate, and hold my clients through these painful healing journeys. Healing is revealing. Our stories can be told in so many beautiful and different ways. I was teaching a new language to clients. Helping them to speak about the unspeakable with words. Most clients could only communicate through the language they had learned through their addictions and chaos. I taught them how to express themselves in new ways. I continued to write more and more and used it in sessions; and the results were profound.

On her next visit I shared the poems with Christine. She sat quietly and listened. As I completed the reading, I felt a sense of peace and gentle, warm energy in the room. Through her tears, she assured me that I understood her and her feelings. I felt a sense of relief and peace as she continued her session that day.

A Year Later

I received a long voice message on my phone one morning. One of the most powerful healing interventions I have used when working with clients with deep trauma and addiction is having them leave a message at any time and talk to me as if in session. This technique has really helped when clients have experienced flashbacks or difficult situations. Usually these clients' tendency would be to use drugs to ease the pain, so in therapy, I encouraged them to call at a later time and talk as if I were present. They would also postpone using when on the phone. Sometimes in the next session, I would replay the message, and we would applaud the effort and the avoidance of drugs or alcohol. Christine used this method many times. After I listened to this particular message, I was inspired to write the following two poems.

She Finally Speaks Her Truth
In a way I am glad we are not meeting today
Over the last few hours in my pain I prayed
The distance between mom and I remains the same
What's new, she called, and so began the game

"Only to check in daughter, only to check in dear"
"We are so separated, so removed; I wish that you were here"
Something inside me began to boil
Confusion, pain, anger, the serpent uncoil

I gathered all my strength in this volcano of feelings
Her, I want to see no more, no more dealings
She neglected me, doubted me, showed me no love
Why all this pain, I ask the Creator above

I waited, took a long breath and then I spoke
At first it was so hard, I thought I was going to choke
I said, mamma, you where never there for me
All your men sexually abused me, I plead

When I showed you my pain, you turned away
I was so scared, I begged you to stay
Mamma, if only you believed me then
I would be a writer, or artist with brush and pen

What can a scared little girl do when Mamma says no!
I felt so dirty, so violated, so ugly, so low
Now you say, it was not all your fault
Where were you Mamma when they entered my vault

You say "stop!" That you cannot take it any more
Hear my cry, the result of the trauma made me so raw
Let me tell you about my life and how I cope
Sometimes I cry, drink, have sex and smoke dope

See mamma all that stuff ease the pain for me
Sometimes in small moments, I feel so free
Then come the past, hurt, depression, resentment and all
Then I am loaded again with fears, tears and I bawl and bawl

I curl up like a baby and wish myself gone
Sometimes I curse the day that I was born
No mamma, the suffering I endured, the pain
How will you ever understand, your denial is a drain
I want you to know that I speak with a lady now
About this darkness, pain, and hurts she teaches me how ...
To love, embrace myself, live and be safe
She rescued me from suicide and grave

See mamma, in this world sisters do care
All of these good things ... do I really want to share?
Mamma, in spite of all my pain, I am still strong
You say I will never make it, but you are so wrong
I am cared for, loved by the Great Spirit you know
Mamma, I am wiser now, I continue to grow

We Hear You Sister, We Hear You

I received your message, I listened
Your call, your hurt, your pain, your plea
I listened, I focused all the way
Right now this is what I need to say

You are so honest, articulate, wise and brave
Those hurtful, raw, painful toxins are now out of the cave
Sister you were the only one who could let them out
Knowing that the healing will take place now, oh I want to shout ...

"She did it, through that fire of emotions, she came!"
From now on things will never be the same
For when we explore our deep hidden wound with open eyes
Some of the demons, the cancers they die

You are women of strength and virtue
To your mission, your calling you are so true
I understand, I feel, I recognize your sorrow
Sleep gentle, peacefully, there is a tomorrow

Full of new promises, gifts, you know
Observing your growth humbly moves me
Thank you for sharing and trusting me so
Those beautiful words about me, I will cherish you know

I am here for you, committed and true
Life you are embracing this new you
I am so proud of you, your courage profound
Listen, can you here in the silence, that beautiful sound?

Comments

Just as the body can be traumatized, so can the spirit and the soul. The term *abuse-related trauma* refers to the wounding of emotions, the spirit, and a will to live. It changes our worldview, our view about ourselves, our dignity, and our sense of security. The assault of the trauma on Christine was so great that her normal ways of thinking about and feeling or dealing with stress became inadequate. Christine was so deeply traumatized that she walked around as if naked and wounded for a very long time.

Christine's Story in Her Own Words

My name is Christine. I am the youngest of five children. My parents got divorced, and my father moved out of the home when I was nine. I was secretly happy about my father's departure until my mother moved her boyfriend into the home soon after.

From the time that I was four to when I was sixteen, inappropriate things were happening to me and around me at home. I told my mother, but she did not believe me or do anything to protect me. The family response was to pretend that nothing was happening, when in my heart I knew that it was. I felt extremely heartbroken, confused, angry, and filled with shame.

I suffered alone with this truth, and up to today my family cannot accept that I was sexually, physically, emotionally, and mentally abused by members of my family and household. The secrets, lies, and family denial were so profound that at the tender age of twelve, I made a vow to myself that when I got old enough to find a job and support myself, I would move as far away from my family as possible and never look back.

My healing journey began at age nineteen when I chose to attend a university far enough away from home that I would have to move and live there. That journey has taken me through abusive relationships, self-mutilation, depression, and addiction. Today at age thirty-eight, I am grieving the end of a five-year relationship. I thought that he was the key to my happiness and a way to help me get distance from my family. I poured myself into doing everything to please him and make him happy.

I know that the healing journey takes its time. I keep in touch with my family because I love them. It hurts to be around them for too long. So, I pick and choose when I want to show up and when it is time to leave. I do not see or speak to my father. My focus today is on learning how to give myself love, support, nurturing, and the respect that I deserved as a child.

Finding the right kind of therapy that works for me has been the key to my healing. I was determined to overcome the darkness that lived inside of me and yearned for a therapist who could relate to me as a black woman. I read self-help books, went through a series of counselors, social workers, support groups, psychiatrists, and psychotherapists until I found Teresa through the Substance Abuse Program for African Canadian and Caribbean Youth, in Toronto. That was when the deep healing began for me.

Teresa got it! She understood my pain and suffering in a way that no other helper before her could. Teresa fearlessly walked through my darkness with me. She believed in me, nurtured my broken spirit. Eleven and a half years later, we are still working together. I have found a mother and a friend for life in Teresa. For this I am truly blessed and grateful.

Conclusion

Part of our role in doing trauma and addiction work is as witnesses. It is with gratitude and with humility that I proclaim the beauty of the spoken word, the art of healing. I began to see and realize that as clients experienced this sacred energy, through validation and support, a profound shift occurred deep within, from an energy that bordered on the miraculous.

The healing power of our hearts can indeed create a chain reaction. When we realize our position and the depth of intimacy with clients and we begin to appreciate this privilege, we begin to transform in this love and connectedness. The connections emerge through acceptance, respect, understanding, love, and compassion. When both client and therapist are transformed by the act of giving and caring, they are nourished by this connectedness. This transformation took place in front of my very eyes. Clients began to recognize, through telling their stories and being courageous, that the healing was far greater and more powerful than their wounds. The act of giving and caring is a reciprocal process or journey.

Chapter Four

Mika's Healing

Introduction

Waiting for Mika, I replayed the words of her doctor. "Teresa, this young person is so in need of your help. If you cannot see her for free, I will pay for the sessions." Those were the words of a deeply caring professional. Mika was thirty-four and had suffered from juvenile diabetes since the age of nine. Despite this hardship and living in a country that could not offer her the best care, she managed to come to Canada at age seventeen and become a psychiatric nurse. As a deeply caring health care professional, it was finally her turn to get the help that she needed.

I walked to the waiting room to meet Mika. There she was: thin, pale, timid. She looked much younger than her age. Her mother was seated right next to her. My first observation was the fear written all over both of them, and it was a sad and painful sight. I introduced myself and asked Mika to follow me to my healing space. Her mother said that she would be waiting for her in the waiting area.

Mika sat down with uncertainty, and I said a few words to make her feel at ease and welcome. I talked about the consultation process and told her a bit about myself. She was quiet and nervous, just listening. When she opened her mouth to speak, her tear ducts opened at the same time, and from then on, her story and struggles were accompanied by tears.

What are tears? A very wise healer once told me that there was no other way to express our innermost, sincere, honest, and gut-level feelings but through tears. This wise women further stated that tears are a gift from the Creator, that we as humans are so fortunate to be able to cry and express the deepest part of our beings.

I reassured Mika and let her know that her tears were good, not a sign of weakness, but of immense strength. She continued to talk about the pain in her heart and all her recent losses. She had had to leave her job because of the progression of her illness. She was in deep grieving and was mourning multiple losses.

In the literature, one will discover that not much has been written on the subject of multiple losses. For example fatigue is described as one of the greatest, hardest losses to cope with.

Fatigue

Fatigue, acute or chronic, is defined as a feeling of weariness or tiredness or a temporary loss of physical and emotional energy to respond to sensory or motor stimuli (Carroll-Johnson, Gorman, and Bush 1998).

In Mika's case this fatigue robbed her of so much more. Her losses were multidimensional. At a physical level she had lost her job; she was unable to perform her daily activities and could not function at any social level. As young woman it affected her sexual functioning and the performance of her duties as a wife and partner. This spilled over into her emotional, spiritual, and mental states. The greatest side effect was that of low self-esteem and self-loathing; she blamed herself and was terribly hard on herself.

Mika felt that she was a burden to her husband and the rest of her family. She felt punished and was suffering at a very deep level.

With all this said, could one take this reality and bring it forth into a positive transformative healing journey? The task would certainly be a challenge, but I do believe that all the knowledge that we possess is not changeless or absolute truth, that we can change our attitude in any circumstance, and when we do that with love and truth, we begin to transform in ways that we never thought possible. This was the case with Mika. Mika's story is about suffering, love, truth, hope, courage, and transformation.

After several sessions and deep healing work, I was inspired to write these two poems.

Multiple Losses

My doctor sent me today to meet with you
She said you are a healer and therapist, is that true?
I am so desperate for healing this day
Many times in my turmoil and sadness I pray

See, I feel that I have lost so much already
The final straw was the loss of my job so steady
I am a nurse so proud of my profession
Why all this suffering, where the lesson?

Pathetic, hopeless, full of sorrow, so helpless I am
I am so young, happily married can you understand?
The darkness, so overwhelming, the pain so great
I doubt that you can help someone in this state

When I was eight, grandpa suddenly died
I loved him so much I was always at his side
My heart broke into little pieces and so
I tried to be brave, no tears did I show

A few weeks later, I was ill and weak
The help of so many my parents began to seek
Diagnosis: Diabetes. My life changed so fast
I was confused, not sure how long it would last
Well, it stayed, and always followed me around
It entered my life, my being without a sound

This thing plagued me, stole my happiness and all
When Mamma prayed, she felt God missed her call
I was no longer to eat all the sweet foods I saw
Just a child, the losses left me angry and raw

My laughter, my joy and all my fun disappeared
Never thought I would have the need to be here
My tears they hurt as I try to fight them away, oh this sorrow
Sometimes I just dread today, yesterday and tomorrow

I have lost so much over the years
Sorry, so sorry, here comes the tears
My health, my body is my wealth no more
Is there hope and healing for this humongous sore?

I want to accept, surrender, live and love
I know in my sorrow that the Creator above
Must have a plan, please help me understand
 I left my country and entered this land

Yes, Canada helped me so much I know
All the gains and the blessings I can show
Healing I need, healing and peace I seek
I've said enough, now it is your turn to speak

Let the Healing Begin

Honored to meet you on this beautiful day
Also hoping that you will decide to stay
Your doctor, so caring, honest and true
Her understanding vast, she advocated for you

I am so moved by your courage and faith
Your heart so big, filled with hope and ache
I see your fear, apprehension, suffering and pain
So much you gave up and what did you gain?

I do not have all the answers you know
As you tell your story our relationship will grow
Trust is what you need the most right now
Let me tell you about the healing journey and how

First step to healing is acknowledgement
My role here is to understand the predicament
This first step is huge for so much you already lost
I made the commitment to help, don't worry about the cost

Safety and self-care will always lead the way
Compassion and caring with practice will stay
Your tears, sadness, pain and suffering so vast
The medication on week four will kick in fast

Your years of struggling took a toll I know
The suffering, fears, pain and tears now show
You are not alone, many loved ones are at your side
Your enlightened witness I am and also your guide

The heart is the place of healing I am so sure
The infinite energy so powerful will cure
All the fears, delusions, pain and confusions
New insight will replace the illusions

No. The why I'll never know, but I'll admit
The questions we sometimes ask of grace and grit
Weak and strong in soul you are here
The mystery the healing so present, do not fear

Meditation, contemplation will open the door
The transformation will leave you in awe
Continue the work, your journey to the light
Persevere as the darkness moves out of sight

Comments

After I shared these poems with Mika, she stared at me in disbelief. In her silence I read, "How could you possibly know all of this about me? How could you possibly understand at such a deep level? How could you possibly know that the interventions you just read about could save my soul?"

"You understand, don't you? You truly do," she said. That was the beginning of trust, understanding, and healing. Mika surrendered.

She let go and accepted things just the way they were then, and something profoundly shifted in the relationship. Two human hearts connected with uncertainty about the future but with hope in the here and now.

Embrace the Mystery

Mika's Story in Her Own Words

My anticipation to meet spiritual healer, Teresa Naseba Marsh, made me feel like I was opening a new chapter in my life. Thank God that both my parents came with me; I was a nervous wreck. Dad drove Mom and me to see Teresa. As the two of us waited in the office seating area, Teresa approached us calmly and politely. *Never in my life have I ever met such a peaceful and spirited person*, I thought to myself the first time I saw her. I felt unbelievable calmness and warmth while shaking Teresa's hand.

When Teresa and I stayed alone in her office, I was speechless. I was trying so hard not to cry, but my body would not listen. Nevertheless, talking with Teresa made me feel good and safe. I was so glad that I finally found the courage to admit that I needed help. I just wanted to breathe again without having all four walls closing in on me at all times.

Why me? Why now? Why is God doing this to me? Those were the questions I frequently asked myself, Teresa, and the universe. As she listened and cared, she told me the following words: "I don't know why this is happening to you right now. Maybe one day you will find out, but at present embrace the mystery of life! Maybe you are asking God the wrong questions. Ask yourself, 'What can I do today to help myself?'" Those words tickled my mind and soul. Thereafter, I began to dig deep into my feelings, actions, and situations around me. Then and there Teresa's words changed my attitude.

The story of Mika began in Serbia. I remember the beginning of my childhood to be extremely happy, eventful, and energetic. This chubby kid loved to eat, dance, and talk. I loved the food my grandma cooked for us. Every bite of her home-cooked meals was a wonderful embrace from heaven. I do not think there was a more chatty little person in the building than myself at that time. Despite being surrounded by kids, I had the most fun with my mom's dad, Grandpa Nikola. The two of us were so mischievous. We used to "steal" money from Grandma's wallet while she was cooking, to go and buy goodies at the store. She would catch us every time, and she would laugh while shaking her head in disbelief. I loved those days.

When I turned eight years old, Grandpa died of a sudden illness. I did not have a clue what death meant, but it felt like my whole world crumbled and disappeared. From then on, I was always afraid death would come and swoop somebody else dear away from me. I wanted to be buried in the ground with Grandpa so I would not miss him so much.

One year after this unfortunate event, I was diagnosed with juvenile diabetes. I was nine years old. Becoming ill felt like I was being punished for something I had done wrong. That feeling of guilt was placed right next to the feeling of punishment. Subsequently, my family was in chaos. I felt like everything was my fault. I pretended like everything was okay or that nothing was wrong with me. This ignorance was truly bliss for me. As soon as I was away from my parents' sight, I took every opportunity not to take care of myself. I smoked, drank, and partied, skipped insulin doses and ate whatever the hell I wanted to. In my mind, I was not worth anything that was good and safe. Even if I understood how necessary good care of my body and soul was, I was too young to accept it. I hated being different from my peers.

It did not help that the general knowledge regarding juvenile diabetes in the eighties was very poor and questionable. The entire issue of properly balancing food, insulin, and exercise at this young age was a truly enigmatic battle. I recollect reading in a book that if a traumatic event occurs before a child forms his or her identity, that same event can cause significant emotional damage to the child. For years, I believed that death would give my body and soul rest. The bed-wetting at night was the worst; I felt a lot of shame. The worst experience was when I peed myself during class in second grade. My blood glucose level was extremely high, and I did not make it to the washroom in time. The whole class laughed, and I was ashamed.

Another difficult thing was going to friends' birthday parties or other types of celebrations. You see, having diabetes follows every aspect of your life; it is not an illness for which you can take your medication and then forget about it. These were some of the thoughts that went through my mind before each celebration: *What will I eat? What will I drink? And what will my friends think of me? Will they tease me? How much can I dance? Will anybody like me? How could anybody like me when I am so different?* Therefore I felt like I lost my childhood and the ability to be carefree. I lost the ability to enjoy food and any celebration because of it. My self-confidence was so severely shaken. I did not have dignity, identity, or independence. *Is there something else I will lose?* I asked myself often.

My luck with peers became better during high school years, before moving to Canada. In 1989 I met my best friend and, today my husband, Sam. First there was a friendship, which turned into love. For him it was love at first sight; on the other hand I could not believe that anybody could love me. When he was told about my illness by one of my friends, he told her that he loved me even more. I could do no wrong in his eyes. Even when I moved to Vancouver at the beginning of the Balkan wars in 1992, we managed to keep in touch via phone and letters. We were apart for four years, and we still loved each other. We wanted to live together, so we married in 1996, at the ages of twenty-one and twenty-two.

In that year, I left school to work a full-time job to sponsor him, and he served the Serbian army to be able to leave the country. When he moved to Canada, we lived with my parents so I could finish the psychiatric nursing program debt-free. During that time my husband worked several different jobs to support my school fees and me. I worked part-time doing home nursing for three years. After the huge amount of emotional and financial support from my parents and husband, I became a registered psychiatric nurse in the year 2000. Being busy working also meant that I could not pay any attention to my health. Caring for people in need gave me the biggest emotional fulfillment but was also the biggest emotional drain. I did not just work as a nurse; I was a nurse to everyone but myself.

As time went by, I became weaker and more ill, which caused a great strain on my work. Because I continued to refuse to see doctors regarding numerous health issues, my marriage became shaky. I felt like a huge burden to my family and husband who worried tirelessly. I was stubborn but also drowning in my own pain and sorrow. I was hopeless and helpless.

In 2004, I was diagnosed with chronic renal failure due to diabetes. My body and my soul became pale, broken, and exhausted. Thus I lost control over my life and my faith for a better future. My husband and I also found out that we were not to conceive a child, under any circumstances, as my body could not go through a pregnancy. When we asked about adoption, the doctors told us not to think about it until my health improved enough. It felt like every additional loss brought me more grief and confusion.

There was more bad news on the way. During one of my visits to Dr. Melamed in 2006, she voiced her concern by stating, "Mika, since your condition is surely brittle and you are getting weaker day by day, I sincerely recommend you stop working immediately. I will speak with your supervisor at the hospital about applying for long-term disability." There went my job and the identity of being a nurse. I felt useless. I felt like my head was hitting a brick wall any way that I turned.

Knowing all the above was happening to me, Dr. Melamed urged me to see Teresa. She said, "If you do not have any money, I will pay for the sessions with Teresa. Mika, to survive the transplant you absolutely have to take good care of your physical and emotional body." My eyes were filled with tears as Dr. Melamed hugged me like only moms do. She also ordered me to write the following on my fridge: "Guilt should not be in any part of your life." So I did.

I wrote it on my fridge. Looking at it, I understood, but I did not accept it yet.

After many tests and interviews at British Columbia Transplant Society, it was decided that my dad would be my kidney donor. My brother could not be considered because of previous treatment for cancer. I felt that I was taking so much out of my loved ones. What could I do in return? "Just take good care of yourself," my loved ones told me. "That will be our biggest gift." The doctors also told me that I was to be considered for a pancreatic transplant later.

Out of all the treatments, I was the most afraid of my hypoglycemic comas. Despite years of taking insulin, my body was very sensitive to it. Poor renal function caused loss of appetite, so even one extra unit of insulin could put me into severe diabetic shock. I was close to death so many times, while my husband and family watched emergency staff work on me many days in a row.

So I asked myself, *Do I allow these losses to beat me, or do I shape up this crazy attitude of mine and face the inevitable—life?*

Mom has always been my guardian angel, so yet again she nudged me in the right direction. I was finally ready to hear her words of wisdom: "Mika, put yourself in your husband's shoes. Would you want to come home from work wondering if your spouse is dead or alive? I worry about you, but there is nothing I can do except talk to you and hope you will hear me one day."

There in the midst of my chaos I started to develop love and compassion toward myself. The love, faith, hope, and compassion represent the depths of my being. I was more spiritual than religious, and now I realize why that was so good for me. In my work with Teresa, she gave me day by day suggestions to follow: embrace the mystery; embrace each day as it is; hope—it will take you to your destiny; your illness is a gift; become childlike; give your deep empathy to others and to yourself; and you are a living angel.

I learned that pain softens a human heart. Suffering enriches your soul by making it compassionate, loving, and genuine. I always believed my illness was a gift and suffering in it made me a better person. Love is giving. Thus, I hope that my story gives faith, love, and compassion to all in need. I became so grateful for all I have in my life. God never makes us carry more than our share. However, we can truly accept that statement if we find what it is that we carry within. Even though losses are many in my life, I did not lose myself. Nevertheless, for every loss, I gained more worthwhile, wise, and healing lessons. I became a better version of myself with all the losses. I asked once why all of this was happening to me. Everything had to happen all at once so I could develop the urge to face it all and survive. If the waves hit you once in a while, you do not feel them as much, but if they hit you one after the other, you become more prone to find strength to break them. My biggest lesson was that with love and the right attitude or a deep look within, I could face any type of battle. There are angels everywhere. Just take a good look.

Conclusion

Dear readers, I just want you to know that all the teachings in the poems came to pass. I do not have the words for it, but know that as I sat in silence with pen and paper, the words moved from a place so deep I call it the love and truth space. It is a place deep and beautiful and a place of knowing that exists in us all. As the days and months went by, we worked together, starting off with deep meditations and contemplations and then sharing stories. Stories filled with sadness, deep pain, deep loss, joy, and laughter. Mika is a very smart and gifted lady; and indeed she challenged me many times. Yes, I would say on everything. That was a good thing; it kept me on my toes. We talked about philosophy, nursing, mental health, addiction, and spirituality—our favorite topic. Through these talks and the telling of stories, I witnessed the insight, the knowing, the acceptance, and the healing in Mika. Mika found the meaning in her suffering, not in days, but in months of sitting together with someone whom she trusted and respected.

One day while I was in meditation, the seven gifts came forth in a vision via my self for Mika. They were:

1. Embrace your mystery.

2. Embrace every day as it is.
3. Embrace hope.
4. Embrace your illness as a gift.
5. Embrace your inner child.
6. Embrace your empathy for others.
7. Embrace yourself as that living angel.

I knew that the minute I gave Mika the information she would challenge me, and she did. It was all good, however, because after that session there was a profound shift in Mika in all the dimensions of her being. Her faith was so powerful that it could move mountains. She possessed a holy and sacred peace that stilled the energy in the room. She knew this, and the smile within her shone through her eyes. She was healed. She still had the diabetes and the kidney failure; she was still awaiting her transplant; and she was still suffering from fatigue. But her soul was healed, and she was at peace. She accepted herself just the way she was day by day in the here and the now. She was now living just the way the great sages described: looking deeply within; being aware of the deeper, truer self; being connected to the infinite and to pure consciousness; and knowing that truth was her identity. I remained the humbled and awed witness. What a gift to be able to witness the life of a living angel.

Chapter Five

Emma Garth

Introduction

Late one afternoon Emma stepped into my office. She was hardly settled in the chair when I sensed that the room's entire energy had changed from joy to deep sadness and pain. It was palpable and visible. Emma appeared tired, exhausted, defeated, very sad, and extremely anxious and apprehensive.

I welcomed Emma into my healing space, introduced myself, and encouraged her to take her time to share what she could on that first visit. She slowly began to share her life story.

Emma was referred to me by her medical doctor. She had been a client of this doctor for over twenty years. She had been referred to me, she said, because her doctor believed that all her problems were related to her deep depression. Over the years, her depression had come and gone, and though she had seen several psychologists, nothing had worked. One psychologist told her that she had a good life and that she should be grateful and get on with it. The second clinical psychologist told her that she had no character, that she needed to get a character, and that he would help her do that over the next several months.

A few days before, Emma told me, she had sat on her bed with a newly filled prescription of sleeping pills, wanting to take her own life. Emma told me she had just wanted it all to stop; she wanted to go to sleep and not have to think anymore. Sitting there, she had begun to think about her two children and what it would do to them. She said she had not thought about the death part, the funeral, and the aftermath; she had just wanted to sleep and for it to all go away.

She was severely depressed. Emma described it as an angel sent from the Creator, her spirituality, and her late mother and grandmother, telling her to think of the children. At that moment she changed her mind. Her doctors started her on antidepressants and encouraged her to set up an appointment with me.

Emma's Initiation into Abuse-Related Trauma

Emma was the oldest of five children: one biological sister and three half brothers and sisters. Her mother had been married three times. Emma's biological father left her mother when Emma was four years old. She remembered that day so vividly. She had loved her dad dearly and begged him to take her with him. He said no to her pleas and left. She never saw him again.

What happened to her at that time? So many painful reactions occurred within her at a physical, emotional, and spiritual level. She became wounded.

At the age of five she was introduced to her new dad. Soon three new siblings joined the family. Emma's memories of being a vulnerable nine-year-old girl were of fights, beatings, shouting matches, and verbal abuse. When she was ill her stepdad would tell her that she was faking it. She could never please anyone and felt like she was a burden to the family and the world. She witnessed her grandfather calling her mother a slut because she had become pregnant yet again. As Emma continued to internalize all this abuse, she became physically ill. She suffered from constant throat infections. Finally she was diagnosed with rheumatic fever when she was thirteen years old and was confined to her room and bed for the next four years. Her high school days were spent with a home tutor and her bedroom walls.

At the age of eighteen she finally stepped out of her house into her first job. Not long after, on August 22, she met James. Three weeks later, they were married. Emma said that she hoped that her parents would tell her not to marry this man. But they did not stop her, and he became her abuser for thirty-seven years. She gave birth to a beautiful son and daughter. They became her support and her reason to survive and live. To date they have been her greatest supports in life.

After several visits I was inspired to write these two poems. As you read the poems, you will begin to understand her story with much clarity. She suffered all her life, and by the time I met her she was suffering from complex posttraumatic stress disorder.

Hear My Plight

I came here today because I decided my lot
I have suffered for too long; hope is all I have got
Left from years of abuse, trauma and pain
I am going crazy; please help me I want to be sane

The last few years took so much out of me
I was cheated, blinded I could not see
In my plight I began to ask the Creator above
To guide me to a healer so that I could love

I was gentle, giving, caring and passive all my life
Is it because I am sick? Why all the strife?
I went from doctor to doctor with the same plea
Only my words, my depression and fear they could see

My soul knew I needed more than a pill
When I asked, they would bid me to be still
Patience. You'll heal continue the medication
They could not hear me, What is the use of conversation?

Fearful nights, painful lonely days I recall
Oh I am so sorry, the tears I am starting to bawl
The tears so painful from a place so deep
Many nights I suffered nightmares and no sleep

Tell me healer where do I begin, is there hope
The last few years of sorrow, hurt I could not cope
Memories come of darkness, sadness of years gone
Why me? Why me? Please tell me what I have done

The last therapist after one session told me that I was weak
Could not help me, he asked, "What do you seek?"
Tears came, confusion, remorse, guilt, I felt so much shame
Again as I left his room, fear, Lord, am I to blame?

Healer please I want to tell my story
I yearn those years I felt peace and glory
I will do the work, but need your direction and wisdom
Please help me, lead me to spirits blissful kingdom

I believe and know deep in my soul there is a light
Now I am embarrassed, am I a pathetic plight?
In this time of my life I should not be in such a place
I feel peace here in your office; I could heal in this space

Comments

During Emma's next visit I shared the first poem with her. As I read she listened deeply, and tears started to roll uncontrollably down her face. She wept in relief. When she lifted her head, her face beamed with hope and courage.

"That's my story," she said. "You know, don't you? You really get it."

This is where the healing starts. We begin to realize that we are not alone anymore, that, yes, the abuse and trauma happened, and that the mind, body, and spirit were deeply injured because of it. The defenses or symptoms that were initiated to help us cope played an important role during the time of injury or trauma. They came into being as a protection for the self. We begin to realize that the defenses persisted and that the ego took all of those wounds on as truth and that the ego is still holding onto those wounds. Those same defenses became a hindrance to our growth and stifled our existence and relationships. The ego will not let go until we wake up, recognize this, and begin the healing journey. In other words, when we become conscious or awake.

It is a fact that healing resides within that therapeutic relationship, deep in the heart of the caring and love that develop between healer and healed. This is what brought about a deep intrapsychic change for Emma. During the healing sessions, she was held, supported, listened to, and validated, and she knew she was safe and acknowledged. Those are the ingredients required for deep healing. Presence—being present in the here and now with another human being—is the medicine, the energy that brings forth deep and powerful insights and thus healing.

Woman with Courage

Your visit today is no coincidence at all
Your faith, determination and hope put out the call
To the universe for help, guidance and direction
Remember after the crucifixion there was a resurrection

Yes woman I see your suffering, struggles and plea
Years of pain, rejection, trauma and betrayal I see
You are here, present, presented, guided today
Your enlightened witness I am so pleased to stay

You say it has been years of verbal and emotional abuse
Looking back at your life, what would you choose?
There in your suffering, fear and darkness you did not know
In your seeking and parenting you started to grow

See, inside of you is your pure spirit, soul, essence your gift
I observe a light in you I sense a lift
Stay with that take deep breaths you are so safe here
Spirit gives light, joy, wisdom and peace, do not fear

First step to healing from trauma is acknowledgement
You have done so; now step two is your commitment
Then we will move within as you tell your story
Believe me slowly you will begin to experience that glory

Comments

A gentle breeze entered the room. The stillness in both healer and client created a safety and energy of deep understanding. I became a witness of the abuse. As I took on the role of witness, Emma was no longer alone or isolated. This process instilled hope, peace, and deep healing.

Emma and I moved forward with the weekly homework of journaling, watching the mind in action, meditation, exercise, yoga, and of course safety, self-care, and reinforcements. The first ten minutes of each session had us sitting together in silence or meditation. During those times she settled into the even deeper part of her being. For the healer it was a time of stillness, to allow the wisdom and guidance from the creative self, the higher self, to come forth. For me it was a time to say to my Creator that I was ready to be the vessel for the powerful medicine that would come forth to continue to heal the client. It was a still time to thank the Creator for the opportunity to present as a witness for another human being; hence I termed the work sacred. The energy and the wisdom that came forth in the sessions were from a higher source, from the force.

Emma's Story in Her Own Words

Many qualified people have written books on fighting and fixing depression. What is depression anyway? Is it tracks that have been laid down in our minds from birth that this is our place in the world? I am writing this with the hope that it might help one person to know that they are not alone in what they are feeling. What they are experiencing is real; the pain they are feeling is real, even though it can't be seen. In sharing my journey with you, I want to tell you about Teresa Naseba Marsh, the most amazing person, who was the answer to my prayers.

Teresa Naseba Marsh, many designations, but just one word to describe her: healer. Teresa once told me simply that I had been wounded. When I arrived for my second session I was given a diagnosis and a prescription, which said "Hear My Plight."

Teresa once told me the heart *chakra* or energy center is the central powerhouse of human energy. It is the mediator between the body and the spirit. It determines the health and strength. The heart center is emotional in nature and helps to propel our emotional development. To be healed means to be fully conscious, to be positive always, to be sure of yourself, and to never need anyone. Obtaining full healing takes hard work and dedication. It will not happen overnight—not next week or next month. It takes patience and time.

All life crises—divorce, death, emotional and physical abuse, abandonment, adultery—have love at their core. The primary strengths of the heart center are love, forgiveness, compassion, dedication, inspiration, hope, trust, and the ability to heal oneself and others. This energy from the heart is the true motivator of the human body and spirit. Love is the purest form of unconditional love.

My story simply put is abandonment, death, emotional, verbal, and physical abuse, adultery, and divorce. My option was one day sitting on my bed with a bottle of ninety sleeping pills just wanting it to stop or believing that my prayers would be answered. I am glad God was listening to my prayers.

There is no magical pill and no short cut to healing. We all have stories that need to be told, acknowledged, worked through, and let go of. We have an ego that does not like to let us forget, an ego that shouts daily, "You are bad! You are bad!" I call it the monster in the box. Two years of hard work, meditation, counseling, prayers, yoga, and healing circles helped me—saved my life. I try not to let the monster out too often, but when he does rear his ugly head, I visualize Teresa's talking stick and put him back in the box where he belongs.

Simply put the Creator will always be there for us. We just need to ask. The gifts are there to receive; we just need to ask and listen. I have learned over the past few years that in the stillness we need to listen.

To achieve consciousness in life, to truly heal, there are no short cuts, and it does not have a timeline. You must do the work. There will be mountains to climb and hills and valleys to overcome. Quite simply put, when going through the healing process, there are ups and downs, highs and lows. Remember, the chatter we hear in our heads is our ego telling and reminding us why we shouldn't do something and the adverse consequences of failing. Remember, that is just the ego trying to keep your mind so small. Use the healing stick; put the ego back in the box.

Self-examination is the first step to personal greatness and healing. Life, our life is such a fragile gift given to us for a relatively short period of time. It is a priceless gift that we have been given to guard and to use to the best of our ability. Our life will not come again; this is what makes it so sacred. The healing journey takes hard work and commitment; however at the end of this journey, life can be extraordinary.

I am now three years into my healing journey. For the first time in my fifty-seven years of life, I know who I am, and I like who I am. I love who I have become. I wrote myself a poem called "Loving Myself."

Loving Myself

Deep at the center of my being
there is an infinite well of love
I now allow this love to flow
to the surface
… It fills my heart,
 my body, my mind,
 my consciousness,
 my very being
Love radiates out from me
every direction
and returns to me
multiplied

I would like to share some thoughts I wrote in my journal during my healing process that put life and the gift that it is in perspective.

Life isn't always fair, but it is still good.
When in doubt, just take the next small step.
Life is too short to waste time hating.
You don't have to win every argument, agree to disagree
Don't compare your life to others; you have no idea what their journey is all about.
If a relationship has to be a secret, you should not be in it.

Thank you, Creator and Teresa, for standing with me during my continued healing journey.

Summary

People stay in broken, abusive relationships for many profound and powerful reasons. Our own brokenness often leads us to others who are broken and bleeding as well. It's like the psyche radar seeks these partners out. But why?

I think Emma describes her reasons for staying so clearly and with deep honesty. When Emma began to understand her illness, her abuse-related trauma, her patterns, thoughts, emotions, actions, and behaviors, something profoundly shifted for her. She could then understand at a very deep level that it was not all her fault. She could then take responsibility for the mistakes she had made.

As she began to understand the ego mind—the monster, as she called it—she gained strength and power to put a stop to the abuse that had continued for so long. She had no need then to be reminded how bad she was, how fat she was, how stupid she was, and so on. She had the power to stop that chatter by living in the present, in the here and now. Indeed she is a courageous and powerful woman who has blossomed into a woman warrior on her own. Emma divorced her husband less than two years after she started her therapy. This work is a process. As we move forward, we allow that process to unfold gently. How do I know that Emma has healed? Very simple: she does not hurt herself anymore.

Chapter Six

Highway to Heaven

Introduction

This story could be any parent's story, yet all parents are unique. Therefore each parent's response to the death of his or her child will be different from that of his or her spouse and other members of the family. There are, however, common responses that will frequently appear at these difficult times. When addiction is part of the picture, the results become even more complex and devastating.

A crisis, especially the death of a child, is accompanied by changed feelings, behaviors, and experiences, coupled with great gushes of a range of emotions, including disbelief, anger, guilt, confusion, and grief. This can be coupled with physical symptoms such as hollowness in the stomach, tightness in the chest, lack of energy, dry mouth, difficulty sleeping, loss of appetite, and frequent crying bouts. Parents become preoccupied with thoughts of their experiences with their children as well as their own childhoods and pasts. Past losses float to the surface, and these memories carry with them pain and suffering. There are intense fluctuations of emotions such as disbelief, anger, and grief. Sometimes these feelings might turn into a sense of powerlessness and loss of control, which can be very frightening.

The Initial Visit

When I met Bonnie in the waiting area, she was accompanied by all of the above emotions and more. Bonnie was the saddest person that I had met in a very long time. The message I received from her doctor was urgent but brief; so everything I was encountering with Bonnie on this day was new. As Bonnie sat down I noticed that she was holding something close to her chest. As I began to ask the usual questions, I noticed a rash on her face and arms.

Bonnie informed me that her doctor had said that she knew someone who could help her deal with her current circumstance and had given Bonnie my brochure. Regarding the rash, she said that she had tried everything but could not get rid of it. When I asked if she had anything stressful happening in her life, she opened the package that she was holding close to her chest and removed a photo of a very handsome young man.

"He should be here in this office today—not me! But it is too late. He is dead!"

I said that I was so sorry about her loss and asked how he died. Bonnie said, "He was addicted to heroin, and he overdosed or killed himself. I am not sure which."

And then the tears came. Along with those words of deep pain and suffering were remorse, guilt, shame, anger, and a host of other painful emotions. I sat in shock with pain in my heart for this mother. What do you say to a mother in this situation? What words could console such deep pain and hurt? I remembered the words I often uttered to young nursing students when I taught them about death and dying: "Nothing you say can make a difference. Just being there and being with them in the most authentic manner is all one can do." So, that is what I did. I sat with Bonnie, and I listened with my heart and held her with my spirit.

Then the questions came. *Why me? Why him? Why us? Why now?* He was so young, such a beautiful, kind human being. *What did I do? What did I not do as a mother? How do I deal with this? Can I heal? Will this ever go away?* The cruelty of it all, the anger with God, and so on—Bonnie questioned it all.

The first session ended with sadness and with reassurance from me as the psychotherapist/healer that it would take time but that we could work together. We had conversations about loss, grief, and, mourning—and especially about self-care for Bonnie, her spouse, and her family. She said that her husband was doing so much better than she was; he was ready to carry on with life. She had only one other child, a daughter, who was sad, but was also carrying on. She felt that she was the only one who could not move forward; she felt stuck and, more so, that she did not want to let go yet. She needed answers to her questions. She needed to find meaning in her suffering.

When her visit with me ended, she did not know if she would return, but she did promise to connect with a phone call.

Comments: Drug-Related Overdoses

Illicit drug-related overdose has been recognized as a common cause of morbidity and mortality among injection drug users (IDUs). In many countries, fatal overdose is a leading cause of death among IDUs, and in response, a variety of overdose interventions have been implemented. In New York City drug overdoses have recently overtaken homicide as the number one cause of death; and in Baltimore overdose deaths increased by more than 425 percent between 1990 and 1997 (Kerr, Tyndall, Lai, Montaner, Wood 2006).

In light of the ongoing harms associated with overdose, several studies identifying the determinants of overdose have been undertaken, with most of these studies focusing on heroin-related overdoses. Among the more consistent predictors of overdose are: polysubstance use (in particular, the concomitant use of central nervous system depressants); a greater number of years injecting; recent release from prison; and injection in public spaces. An array of overdose prevention interventions have been initiated, with most of these initiatives focusing on educating drug users about the risks of overdose. However, the limitations of education-based prevention programs have been highlighted, with critics suggesting that these programs fail to consider the social and contextual factors that drive risks such as polysubstance use.

Second Visit

Bonnie came back to see me. She said that after her first visit she felt some sense of relief for the first time. She saw changes in some of her symptoms and a slight improvement with the rash.

This second session was dedicated to Bonnie sharing information about her son, their life, how he had grown up, and their frequent travels to different parts of the world due to the nature of her husband's business. She talked about her role as a parent and mother, specifically, and looked deeply into herself, trying to figure out where she had gone wrong. She felt deeply that it was her fault, that she had not done enough as a mother. She thought that she and her husband, as a couple, had not handled the situation correctly when they discovered that their son was addicted to heroin. She was angry at the system and felt that the system had failed them. She talked about how they had been sent from pillar to post.

The saddest part of it all was that it was not until after the death of her son that she met Dr. Jenny Melamed, the referral doctor, who was a specialist in addiction medicine. She found Jenny to be very knowledgeable and smart and believed that Jenny could have saved her son. She said, "And now I meet you. He would have benefited from seeing you, a spiritual healer."

She shared a bit with me about his character and how he talked about the spiritual realm and paranormal experiences that he often had. Often, he felt misunderstood. From what she shared with me, Cameron sounded like he was an indigo child.

During this session, we also talked about the process of mourning and the tasks involved.

The Tasks of Mourning

Task One: Accept Reality

When someone dies, even if the death is unexpected as in Cameron's case, there is always a sense that it hasn't happened. The first task of grieving is to come to full face with the reality that one's child is dead and gone and will not return and that nothing will be the same again.

Part of accepting of reality is coming to the belief that reunion is impossible, at least in this life. Many people who have sustained loss find themselves calling out for those they have lost, and they sometimes mistake others in their environment for their loved ones out of a desire to see them alive once more. This experience is described as searching behavior. This can be a very trying time coupled with tremendous pain as the parent realizes more and more that his or her child is truly gone.

Bonnie's Process and Journey

This was a very difficult and painful task for Bonnie. She had so many unanswered questions, and her disbelief and guilt always came to the fore. She dealt with this by almost punishing herself. She always talked about what she did not do and so on. She neglected herself and the things that used to bring her pleasure. Her family was very concerned. We examined her life often, but it was difficult for her to move forward.

We started off the sessions with sitting together in meditation. After the silence I was distracted by a presence and a voice that kept on telling me to tell his mother that he was in the room and had a message for her. I was not going to cooperate because I felt Bonnie would not understand or accept this. I said no, but he persisted.

He described a shirt that he used to wear at home and asked me to describe it to her to help her believe me. I still said no. He persisted and said that it was important, that she would understand, and that I should trust him.

Bonnie noticed that I was distracted and asked me what was going on.

"Your son is here," I told her as his presence overwhelmed me. She rubbed her arms as she stared at me, tears rolling down her face. I thought she might leave.

"What is the message?" she asked.

"He loves you very much, and it was nobody's fault. He is an angel now. It was his time to go home, for he had other work to do. His time on Earth was done."

Bonnie nodded her head in understanding.

"He's at peace and wants you to continue on with your life. Celebrate."

Bonnie smiled.

"Oh, and I am supposed to mention his special brown shirt with button-down pockets. Does that mean anything to you?"

Tears streamed down Bonnie's face as she cried in relief. "Thank you," she said. At the next session she brought in the shirt to show me.

That experience helped Bonnie to fulfill this first task. She began to say yes to life and take good care of herself. As the weeks went by I noticed changes in the colors she wore, just small, beautiful changes. I began to sense her peace. She began to share stories of feeling his presence in her house and garden. Her eyes lit up as she spoke.

Healing is a long journey that requires time and patience. Each person's journey is unique.

Task Two: Work Through the Pain and Grief

This is indeed a painful journey, and it is experienced physically, emotionally, and behaviorally. It is necessary to acknowledge this pain and work through it, or it may later be expressed in different, more complicated ways. This is not easy in the least; often parents describe it as unbearable and overwhelming, something that eats away at them. At this time they also have to cope with loved ones and friends who might want to help remove the pain as soon as possible. Sometimes others who find it extremely difficult to see parents' suffering might even minimize the pain, urging a mother or father to get over the pain as soon as possible. Some people do this by stimulating only pleasant thoughts of the deceased, which protect them from the discomfort of unpleasant thoughts.

As I said in the introduction, this element was hard for Bonnie. She experienced all of the above, and when family members told her to accept her son's death, she was laden with guilt and shame. During our sessions she worked through this via storytelling. She talked about the unpleasant events that had occurred as well as the pleasant ones.

One of the most painful memories she shared was of the time when Cameron had been in a treatment center but had left after deciding that it was not for him. The center called Bonnie and told her not to take her son in. She asked me how anyone could ask that of a mother. She totally understood that Cameron could not relate to the people and the type of therapy they offered him. The center had also encouraged him to go off his methadone, and he was in withdrawal. Bonnie took him in, and while they waited several days to get him back into a withdrawal management center, they had to go to his previous dealers to get the medicine to help him through the withdrawal.

They were so lost and did not know where to turn for help. As she educated herself about his addiction, Bonnie realized that Cameron had tried to quit many times. In addition, she saw the withdrawal but did not know what it was. Her husband, a very realistic and practical man, dealt with the situation in a more practical, intellectual manner. I had the sense that as Bonnie healed and shared our sessions with him, he was vicariously healed as well.

Task Three: Adjust to the New Environment

Not only do parents have to adjust to the roles played by their children, but they also are confronted by having to adjust themselves. *Who am I now?* parents ask. Recognizing that one's nurturing role has been taken away is a frightful and painful realization. Bereavement can also lead to intense regression during which the bereaved perceive themselves to be helpless, inadequate, incapable, childlike, or personally bankrupt. This experience can also change a parent's sense of the world; fundamental life values and beliefs about many things can be challenged. Some people just withdraw from the world for a while.

It was clear that Bonnie had moved through all of this. The day she came into my office, clutching the picture of her son, she looked like a little girl lost in pain and full of fear. But as the months went by I got to know the most intelligent, compassionate, spiritual, and caring person.

Task Four: Release and Move On

Bereaved parents often have difficulty understanding the notion of emotional withdrawal. This task is about continuing to live with the memories of one's child and having an ongoing relationship with those memories but at the same time continuing on with life.

One of the most painful stages that Cameron's parents went through was feeling as though they had not given enough or had not done all they could. During this time the Canadian Society of Addiction Medicine Conference was being held in Vancouver, and I decided to invite Bonnie and her husband to attend. It was a shot in the dark, but I felt that it was worth stepping out of the box in this situation. My husband, Dr. David Marsh was the president of the society at that time. I just asked him if we could make an exception and allow this couple to attend the conference. He wanted to know why. I said that they had many unanswered questions and that I believed that this scientific conference would help them tremendously on their healing journey. With that, it was done, and indeed it did help them. They met addiction specialists from all over the provinces and began to appreciate the complexity of this problem and more so what was being done about it. This was the most precious gift they could ever have received. It was healing and revealing. I will let Bonnie tell you herself in her story.

Bonnie also had many other deep spiritual experiences and enlightened moments with her late son that helped her a great deal. She once stated in one of our sessions, "Of late I have noticed that life—and the universe in her own sweet way—offer me beauty in spite of the pain. I am beginning to appreciate my garden, the budding of new flowers, the sunrise and sunset, the mountains— and sometimes I see Cameron's face in it, smiling at me, and letting me know that everything is exactly the way it should be. Sometimes I sense a feeling of warmth in his room; sometimes it is almost bittersweet. I am beginning to notice that I am doing much better at tasks; I can complete and enjoy things more. Sometimes I just see Cameron standing over there, watching, smiling, and then I realize that I am still alive, and I am carrying on living as he told me. I just take it one day at a time. It really and truly gets better all the time. I have all his memories, right here in my heart. They will always be ours. I am his mother."

Letter from Bonnie

November 27, 2009

Teresa Naseba Marsh
Psychotherapist/Healer/Educator
Vancouver, B.C.

Dear Teresa,

Thank you for inviting me to contribute to your upcoming healing book about enlightenment.

The painful emotions of the loss of my son five years ago, the horrifying disease of addiction and the pathway to well being are locked somewhere between my mind, my heart, and my soul.

Teresa, to get through all the layers of protection around my heart, I found I couldn't use a pseudonym for my son's name. Couldn't get in touch with my feelings and felt as if I was hiding: cowardly and ashamed. If Cameron's name needs to be changed for publishing purposes, could you please do it for me? I know you will understand.

As the title of this chapter is "We Lost Our Only Son to Heroin", I felt strongly our son would want his voice heard. I have included two of his poems and some of his written thoughts.

Cameron awakened me to the torment of the terrifying disease of addiction and I hope my personal story written from the heart will be read from the heart. That it will bring some awareness of the disease and demonstrate that through all the hope and all the hopelessness of addiction love continues to grow and even grows stronger.

Thank you for this opportunity, Teresa.

Bonnie

Bonnie's Story in Her Own Words

I often had conversations in my mind with my son after he died. Talking to him is a way I seem to be able to locate my feelings and relate my dark journey from shattering despair, unfathomable loss, and terrible confusion toward an enlightened journey of understanding, elated happiness, and transformed spirituality.

I find myself dividing my son's twenty-nine years in two parts: Before addiction and after addiction.

Before Addiction

I remember you sitting at the kitchen table writing a poem and so proudly handed it to me. Your grade eleven English teacher at school had written in your report card: "Cameron demonstrated an emerging personal voice and style. Another literature teacher compared your writing to Roald Dahl. I thought that was ironic because you never wanted me to read his books to you.

Have the trust of a human heart
Fury of doubt
To decide upon
What should it be?
That tips the scale of equality.

Share to a family
Be part of a community
Live harmoniously in society
Be looked up for security

Joke and play and never be apart
Share this joy
A blond haired blue-eyed son
Make life full.
And employ total responsibility.

We had fun as a family, we laughed, we sang, we worked together, cried together. There was nothing to suggest the looming battle of addiction lay ahead.

After Addiction

Cam, you knew, my brave son, you faced the battle alone for so long until we realized the disease had knocked at our door and invited itself in.

The demon in my mind spoke
Echoing in its chamber
Come on, go on, take a toke
Lost
Join my slumber

He drilled
And filled
Me
With ideas which almost
Killed me.

His clamp and clutch
Grabbed my soul
Reality I could no longer touch
My pupils black holes.

He had me hard hold
My spirit to him I sold.
Now zombied in thought

I'm addicted and caught
Following, wherever I stop
With his Hades of death
I have been shot

I reread a note you sent from a drug treatment center to me: "To become a mother is not hard. To be a mother is."

I wrote back, "I loved raising my children, I wouldn't have wanted to do anything else." I knew you meant *to be the mother of a drug addict.*

Folly of youth, you told us. Addiction? What's that? It pained me to the core to read from your journal. You wrote, "I feel like I'm my own understudy of stupidity." It's an unjust disease, my love.

With tears flowing, I read in one of your journals how elated you were when the road to health seemed so close:

After all I'd seen and questioned all that was bewildering, all that was lost and all that was accomplished, I decided to sit down and spell it all out on a pad of lined paper.
The emotional roller coaster ride is not part of the ingredients for my next journey. Exploration of self-destruction had brought me to addiction and the brink of death, but I still carried my head high and with blinded focus all I could see was the future and what joyous adventures stood ahead on my highway of life.
I had met some of the most care giving loving people that inhabit this world and that includes my own family. All the ropes and tethers that bind my family have been made stronger, wiser and in the end a more beautiful picture than ever before.
Back on track with no dangling carrot, no dependency, other than the beauty of life itself, I strive ahead to search for more and for more new meanings.

My beautiful son, although addiction has been around since recorded history, you were born too soon. It is the dark ages for this disease.

After you left, I was broken. We were all broken, and I sought help. Teresa Marsh became my healer and through me the healer of your dad. She listened when I wept and said I had to experience your pain, your loss. I had to feel your soul before I could go through my own nightmare of brutal realization.

As I look back, Cam, I was trying to keep you. Teresa understood I was not ready to "let go." I was not ready to let you slip away into memory. In the warmth of her profound, understanding presence and her deep spirituality, she let me keep you until I was ready to start my agonizing journey of grieving.

Healing through storytelling, Teresa learned about our beautiful family and all about you. Teresa also told her stories. The stories brought me relief from an excruciating endless darkness and screamingly terrifying pain and I wanted to stay in those stories.

Every week I kept getting stronger. I no longer felt like I was going crazy. No longer had the frightening impulse of running, running away and disappearing into infinity. I felt like I was being called and knew exactly which way to go. I guess I hadn't actually crossed over into insanity, Cam, because I knew.

Even my neighbor, Mary, would stop me. "What's happening?" she'd ask. How could I explain I was running into infinity?

The mysterious skin rash started to disappear. *Better the rash disappearing than me*, I can laugh now. You were the comedian in the family, Cam. We were relieved to find we could still laugh as a family when you left.

Teresa patiently listened as I tried to explain the complex emotions we as a family had to work through. My husband had also lost his son, my daughter had lost her brother, and my daughter-in law had lost her husband.

I felt I was a burden on them. My husband didn't suffer the guilt, anger, or shame as I did. After some initial questioning, he knew he had given all his love and all the help he was capable of giving to our son.

I started glorifying you, and your sister would keep me in reality. "He wasn't that good. Remember all the worrying? Teasingly, she'd add, 'He always was your favorite child.'" Who would have thought sibling rivalry would continue after death?

My gorgeous daughter-in-law and my son shared a love that seemed like they were going to kiss the sky. They also experienced stress in the marriage when Cam was actively using. Their arguments were always about his drug use. They had separated but reunited after he entered a treatment center. I was healing from his death through storytelling and she wanted to run away. At a healing circle Teresa initiated, I met a young woman who had lost her husband, and listening to her story helped me understand Linda's feelings of abandonment.

I kept agonizing with Teresa, a substance abuse counselor, over what I should have done, what I should have changed, what went wrong. What is the meaning? What is the reason of your death?

She knew you had awakened me to a medically neglected disease that kills. I was angrily frustrated that anyone thought they could have a medical opinion about addiction. Many sessions were spent with me obsessing about what was or wasn't being done about the disorder.

I talked about the dehumanizing of people with drug abuse disorder, lack of facilities for treatment, the dial-a-drug system, criminals not patients, the demeaning language of clean and dirty, the disconnect of the health system, and the disagreement among professionals as to what is the best treatment, the "Let's get hard on drugs" thinking that held considerable clout. "There is a pandemic," the coroner told us. She explained that she had seen too many young people die from overdosing. Cam, the narrow-mindedness, wasted lives and death still continues.

Teresa arranged through her husband, David Marsh, president of the Canadian Society of Addiction Medicine in 2005, for your dad and me to attend the upcoming conference in Vancouver. Listening to the latest scientific and medical information from professionals and the knowledge that there were dedicated people working on better treatment and a cure helped to put me at peace.

I don't obsess anymore, but I try to keep up on the latest information about addiction.

Thanks to Teresa I knew I could continue on my own. I had a garden waiting to be tended that in turn would tend to me. A loving home. Joyous bundles of love—my grandchildren. Family and friends were waiting. I felt the warmth of the sunshine. I was climbing out of a black hole and into the light. I could be happy. There were still shadows, Cam; but as you know, there are always shadows, and that's not a bad thing.

And thank you for helping, Cam. We all miss very much your healing touch. How I prayed you could heal yourself. In one of my desperate moments I suddenly had a flashback. Do you remember when you came home from a college psychology course and explained the class had done an exercise grading parenting skills? You smiled and said, "You guys had come at the top of the class." Then you paused and looked at me and said, "If you're the best parents, why aren't I the best son?" We pondered the thought then laughed. The word addiction was still eleven years away.

You know me. I said no to sleeping pills, Valium, or anything else. Well, I have to tell you about the wonderful feeling of gold-sprinkled warmth that slowly flowed from my toes to my head on one of my sleepless nights after you died. I know there's probably a reasonable explanation, but I like to think it was you helping me and educating me on the power of your drug of choice: heroin. It was wonderful; I never slept so well. It never happened again. Where have you been?

It's almost Christmas and time for a Christmas story. After you died, our friend Kathy told me the story of the two of you discussing the possibilities and your ideas and enthusiasm for starting a charity fund at her annual Christmas party instead of guests bringing gifts for her. I knew your disappointment when she said she just couldn't do it because collecting money from friends felt uncomfortable.

Cam, your idea for a raffle was fantastic. Kathy said she was disappointed in herself, but in your memory she was going to do it.

It's not as exciting as your plans, but money and clothes have been collected and donated to worthy causes every Christmas since your passing. Merry Christmas!

We donated and planted a big, bold tree in your memory. There's a story, but it's for another time.

Kathy was visiting the garden recently (must have been at your herb garden) and came back into the house with wide eyes and a surprised smile.

"Cameron's in the garden," she gasped. "I'm not kidding. I felt him."

I smiled back and quietly said, "I know."

I thought you must have checking out the veggie garden and fruit trees that you and my dad had relentlessly pushed me to plant last year. You guys ganged up on me. You always said, "Flowers are pretty, but you can't eat them." I kept telling your dad, "There's a strong energy pushing me to get this garden planted. I have to get it planted!"

There's good news in the dreadful world of addiction. An article says it's theoretically possible to take kids before their first drink and find out if there are any gene variations. Wouldn't that be wonderful to have a head start and be ahead of the disease?

I have let go, Cam, but sometimes I cheat. My favorite dream is to see you walking to a local clinic for your medication. No drama or questions as to what medication you are taking—no different than a diabetic receiving insulin. The clinic could be called Insite.

I can hear you, Cam. I can hear you saying, "C'mon, Mom, it's time to go. Your life is with the living; and you have your work, and I have mine. I love you. Ta-ta." I love you.

Conclusion

There is a sense in which mourning can be finished, when a person regains interest in life, appreciating that sunrise, sunset, or first snowfall, experiencing some pleasures again, and adapting to new roles.

All of the coping strategies and defense mechanisms discussed in this chapter are indeed real, present, and absolute. We can't go under the trauma or loss, or over it; we have to go through it. During the painful journey, telling the story of your loss is the most important vehicle to ultimate healing. Every death creates a story (or a set of stories) to tell. Each story has a beginning, with a diagnosis, as well as shock, disbelief, fear, pain, anger, and the unknown. The middle contains experiences, suffering, pain, growth, and uncertainty. The story concludes with events leading up to the death and the experiences of family members. A story captures a series of emotional events and helps us to achieve mastery of those events. So it was in Bonnie's case. We sat together so many times, through the stories she and I both told.

Tell your stories, for in them lies the key and path to emotional relief. Story telling helps to make experiences meaningful and bearable. It provides the answers to why, and it brings understanding and unites people so that healing can occur. The entire purpose of this book has just been described. May all of these stories shared and read be that elixir, the balm that the world so desperately needs today.

Chapter Seven

Concurrent Disorders

Introduction

Addiction and mental health are linked, as already discussed in the previous chapters. Psychiatric and addiction problems are often accompanied by many kinds of complex psychiatric disorders, most frequently, schizophrenia. Mood disorders, anxiety disorders, posttraumatic stress syndrome, and personality disorders are also common.

A wide variety of psychoactive substances can be abused alone or in combination. These include stimulants (e.g., amphetamines, caffeine, cocaine, and nicotine), sedatives (e.g., alcohol, barbiturates, benzodiazepines, and inhalants), narcotics (e.g., heroin and morphine), and hallucinogens (e.g., cannabis, LSD, PCP).

The symptoms of one condition may mask the symptoms of the other—or even make them worse. This is one of the toughest challenges health care professionals face. Being aware and knowledgeable about the complexity of both disorders gives professionals a better chance of helping and supporting people on the road to healing and recovery. Some people might present with one disorder dominating the clinical picture. If the concurrent nature of their problem is not known or understood, however, these clients may find that, after becoming sober, their moods remain low or their anxiety or anger persists.

I hope Kevin's story, told in this chapter, will shed light on the importance of the diagnosis and treatment of multiple disorders existing concurrently in one person. Before he entered therapy with me, Kevin had fallen through the cracks many times; and he was about to give up by putting himself in dangerous situations. This acting-out behavior can also be viewed in the context of crying out for help, a topic covered in the discussion of repetition compulsion or reenactment. The sad part is that, when Kevin placed himself in these dangerous situations, he could have lost his life. In his confusion about what was really wrong with him, he became despondent and in effect tried to commit slow suicide.

The Beginning

What brought Kevin to me was yet another one of his acting-out episodes. He was twenty-three years old and had met up with a girl who was abusing cocaine and cannabis. They had known each other for just two weeks when Kevin decided to give up his place and move in with her. It was a disaster from the word go. They spent all day just getting high. Cannabis was Kevin's substance of choice, but in his acting out, he sought other drugs like LSD, mushrooms, and so on. His major problem at that time was his anger. When Kevin was high—no matter the drug—he would become blindly angry. But this time he had chosen a girl who also had an anger issue. One Sunday night they had a huge fight. His girlfriend won the fight and kept Kevin hostage at knifepoint. The neighbors called the police, and Kevin's life was saved yet again. But in the process he lost all his expensive electronic equipment; he was into computers and the technology used to create music with pictures for raves. He was devastated and of course traumatized yet again by the experience. Fortunately, Kevin's girlfriend had given him my card at one point, so he decided to call me.

First Contact

Kevin showed up at my office a week after the incident in shock and disbelief. He repeated the details of the incident to me and said that he had flashbacks and nightmares; he could not believe that he was still alive. At that time he exhibited symptoms of posttraumatic stress syndrome and was also preoccupied with thoughts of killing himself. He stated that he had walked in front of cars a few times, but nothing had happened. He was deeply remorseful for his behavior and said that he was so tired of not getting it right. He had struggled all his life, and all he wanted to be was a good person. He admitted to still smoking cannabis heavily. He was also using other stimulants (from what I could tell, LSD and mushrooms). He really wanted to stop his drug use, but his attempts to quit had always failed.

I allowed Kevin to tell his story and just listened with all my heart and supported him throughout. He talked about his paranoia and his sadness and related it to the traumatic event with his girlfriend. At the end of this session I talked to Kevin about concurrent disorders and PTSD. I explained to him that he had been retraumatized and that his entire being would need deep caring and support on his healing journey. During this session we developed a therapeutic alliance; and he appeared quite ready to embark upon his healing journey. At the end of the session I told Kevin that he would have to try to stay off the drugs so that I could do a proper assessment and help him appropriately. He agreed, and we scheduled weekly sessions.

Childhood Background

On his next visit Kevin reported that he had used much less than normal in the time since our first session but admitted to having had a joint here and there. He appeared to be more relaxed and more connected. He shared his tragic life story with me. He was born to two young parents, free spirits who both used alcohol and drugs. He described his upbringing as severely traumatic. His mother suffered from a severe mental illness, and his father was heavily into drugs.

His memories of his childhood were scattered, but on this day he talked about his early years and his abusive relationship with his mother. She would beat him endlessly, and he could not understand why. She always told him that he was a naughty child. Many nights he was left on his own and went to bed with no supper.

72

He remembered that his mother was always angry with him. As he recalled these memories he said that, in spite of this, he loved his mother and missed her a great deal. He had few memories of his father but described him as gentle and kind. His father's parents were the stable couple in Kevin's life, and he spent many days and nights with them. He adored his grandparents.

His father, who was a heroin addict, often hung out on the downtown eastside. When Kevin was twelve years old, his father died from an overdose of heroin. Kevin was devastated, and his mom had a breakdown. Not too long after that, he was taken into custody and moved in with his foster parents. He talked fondly of his supportive foster parents, and the next seven years appeared to be stable. He did well in school, although he described going through a stormy adolescence characterized by acting-out behavior. He became involved in acting and did very well with it.

At the age of nineteen he was making a lot of money, and he owned his own apartment and a car. He described the next few years as "party time." He just wanted to have fun and party with his friends. He began using cannabis habitually and said that it calmed him. His drug use increased, and he experimented with multiple drugs. He fell into a downward spiral and lost everything.

He talked about this with deep sadness and regret. He wept as he described a deep, empty sadness. One of the events in his life that gave him strength and stability was some part of his schooling. He had attended a First Nations School and was deeply influenced by the community's spirituality. He befriended an elder during that time, and it appeared as though that contact influenced him deeply.

Kevin had a deep compassion and understanding for humanity, especially the marginalized, and he spoke out with honesty about oppression and racism. He told me that he really enjoyed the First Nations' spiritual teachings. I shared with Kevin some of the work I did in the First Nation communities, and during that session he asked me if we could smudge (make brushings with sage) to remove all the negativity from him. We did. He also requested that we do a healing circle in one of his sessions. We did, and it was profound; from then on, he embarked upon a deep healing journey.

During the next sessions, which focused on history taking and observations, it became clear that Kevin suffered from complex posttraumatic stress disorder coupled with an addiction to cannabis. We talked about this at length and utilized psychoeducational strategies throughout all the sessions. Kevin was encouraged to stay off all drugs, and one day he asked me to set up a written contract with him. We did, and it took him into another level. We began to plan his treatment.

Stage One: Engagement

This stage is initiated when dually disordered clients enter treatment. The goal of engagement is to form a trusting relationship, or working alliance, which enables the clinician to support the client through the substance addiction treatment. A number of interventions may facilitate the engagement process: practical assistance, empathic interviewing, crisis intervention, and forming an alliance with family or social network members. Most of these grow out of the validity of the client's worldview. Here the clinician works collaboratively with the client and implement the strategies that work best for him or her.

In Kevin's situation, we identified what had worked for him in the past as we focused together on the present. Many sessions were used to deal with yet another crisis that came up, after a rave and weekend bender, for example. He was depressed, a fact that became clearer as he stopped using completely. The symptoms of PTSD walked with him, and he would have great days and really bad days.

We talked about antidepressants. Kevin was very connected with his doctor, which was a blessing. This doctor had delivered him as a baby and was a father figure in his life. He was very supportive and made sure that Kevin stayed on his antidepressants. We also set up a family meeting with Kevin's foster parents. They were an amazing, supportive couple and loved Kevin dearly. By this time Kevin was back in his own apartment and was working. He reconnected with his grandparents also, who were his role models. They loved and supported Kevin too.

Things were looking up. As Kevin became clean and sober, he focused on his spirituality. We started off the sessions with grounding, centering, focusing, and meditation. This really helped him. He carried out his weekly homework assignments, which consisted of keeping himself safe, engaging in self-care, focusing on good nutrition, tracking his thoughts, dealing with his anger, and staying clean and sober. This stage of the treatment involves embracing acceptance, expressing empathy, listening carefully, reflecting the client's views back, and understanding.

Kevin was doing well but had one deeply rooted problem: his anger. We spent many sessions dealing with his anger. He was working in construction at the time, with men from all walks of life. Some were aggressive and verbally rough. Kevin struggled in those relationships. He would often speak up to defend himself, but the outcome would be a fight. Kevin had difficulty in letting things go, because his inclination was always to make things right. We started working diligently on anger management, but his temper remained a thorn in his side.

About Anger

We all know what anger is, and we've all felt it, whether as a fleeting sense of annoyance or as full-fledged rage. Anger is a completely normal, usually healthy, human emotion. But when it gets out of control and turns destructive, it can lead to problems—at work, in personal relationships, and in the overall quality of one's life. And it can make a person feel as though he or she is at the mercy of an unpredictable and powerful force. It is one of the debilitating symptoms of PTSD

Anger is "an emotional state that varies in intensity from mild irritation to intense fury and rage," according to Charles Spielberger, PhD, a psychologist who specializes in the study of anger. Like other emotions, it is accompanied by physiological and biological changes; when you get angry, your heart rate and blood pressure go up, as do the levels of your energy hormones, adrenaline, and noradrenaline. Anger can be caused by both external and internal events. Worrying or brooding about your personal problems can cause anger. Memories of traumatic or enraging events can also trigger angry feelings. In Kevin's case, both of these factors were at play.

The instinctive, natural way to express anger is to respond aggressively. Anger is a natural, adaptive response to threats; it inspires powerful, often aggressive, feelings and behaviors, which allow us to fight and to defend ourselves when we are attacked. A certain amount of anger, therefore, is necessary to our survival. But we can't physically lash out at every person or object that irritates or annoys us; laws, social norms, and common sense place limits on how far our anger can take us. In Kevin's case it was all of the above.

We worked together on his anger in session after session. Kevin lost several jobs because of his anger and misunderstandings, but he never gave up.

Stage Two: Persuasion

When a working alliance is formed, the clinician begins to help a client to develop motivation for an abstinence-oriented intervention. The goal is to prepare the client for active change strategies. This can only be done through collaboration with the client and by looking deeply at his or her personal needs and preferences.

Kevin was on the right track and sailed smoothly through this stage. He was so proud to be clean and sober and talked at length about the beautiful changes he had begun to observe in himself. He still had a problem with friends from his past, people he had used with. During this time he would bring difficult and challenging weekend episodes to the session, and he began to understand his patterns and behaviors so much better. He was taking good care of himself, but he still struggled with anger.

Stage Three: Active Treatment

After several months of exposure to persuasion-stage interventions, most clients adopt the goal of abstinence and are ready for active strategies. As you can see in Kevin's case, he was way ahead of the game. He was highly motivated, very intelligent, and involved in his world. He would come to sessions and inform me about what was happening in different parts of the world. He had a vision and dream to help the world heal. He had deep empathy for those who were needy, poor, and suffering and expressed this with heartfelt honesty.

Sometimes we would just engage in storytelling. He loved my stories about others who had come for healing and always wanted to know how they had healed. He often expressed his fondness for me at the end of sessions and would say that he was so lucky to have such a powerful spiritual healer.

Stage Four: Relapse Prevention

Once the client has been sober for six months, treatment focuses on relapse prevention. During this stage Kevin and I talked a lot about the possibilities of relapse, not just with regard to drugs, but also concerning the trauma work Kevin was engaged in. We looked at ways to keep Kevin safe, and he was engaged in the process. One day, a year after his first meeting with me, he cancelled the session. He had lost his job again and told me that he could not afford the sessions any longer. He said that he had plans to go back to school and embark upon more interesting things.

I offered to see him pro bono, but Kevin declined, saying he was too proud. He promised to check in with me from time to time because he realized that his work was not complete. We agreed. Over the next year I received a few phone calls from Kevin, and he reported that he was doing well. He was working again and had met a beautiful girl. He said that she was an English language student from Japan. He sounded happy and content, but he had also relapsed heavily into smoking cannabis. He did not disclose this to me himself; I received a call from his girlfriend,

Hannah. During that conversation I encouraged her to ask Kevin to continue seeing me.

The Crisis Call

This call came a few months after Hannah first contacted me. In her broken English she told me that Kevin was in prison for assault. They had been on Grouse Mountain hiking. He was smoking a lot of cannabis and was suspicious. The events that followed happened very fast, but she remembered Kevin saying that he thought the men behind them were watching Hannah. He stopped and confronted the men, and a huge fight erupted. The police came and arrested Kevin for assault with a dangerous weapon.

I later received a call from Kevin. He was angry, scared, and fearful and sounded like he was psychotic. He was transferred to a psychiatric inpatient facility in Vancouver. He wanted to go home but remained angry and argumentative. As a result he ended up in solitary confinement; he remained alone in a dark room under heavy sedation.

Days later I received another call from Kevin, asking me to visit him in the hospital. He wanted to go home but feared that he would end up in prison. He said that he needed to talk about his experience and tell his side of the story. I agreed to see him and then called ahead to ask his nurse if I could share some of my information with the psychiatrist.

Hannah told me that Kevin had been diagnosed with schizophrenia and was heavily medicated. (In her country, Hannah had been a pharmacist.) Hannah had also shared in Kevin's heavy cannabis smoking behavior over the past few months. She said that he had also been using other drugs, but she was not sure which ones; and she explained that she thought he was depressed.

On my arrival at the unit, Kevin greeted me dressed in hospital pajamas. He was embarrassed and said that he just wanted to have his own clothes. He sat me down in his calm manner and told his side of the story. Then he talked about his diagnosis and said his doctors had already told him that he has to take the medication all his life. He said he had told the psychiatrist about his work with me and would appreciate it if could speak to him.

I went to the nurses' station, and through the glass I saw the nurse and psychiatrist. I stood there for a while and got the nurse's attention. When she came out she told me that she had already told the psychiatrist that I was Kevin's therapist and wanted to share some information him. The psychiatrist had said that he did not have the time to talk to me. I asked her if we could set up a time. She looked at me but did not answer; I got the message.

I stood at the glass window for a while longer. The nurse joined the psychiatrist back at the station; and I watched them talking, but neither of them looked up or even acknowledged me standing there. I was shocked and very confused by their treatment of me. I left and went back to Kevin's room. Kevin wanted to know what the psychiatrist thought. I told him the truth.

I then traveled back downtown with Hannah, feeling devalued, confused, and disrespected. Hannah observed my disappointment and told me that she felt that same way. Nobody had spoken to her or asked her for collateral. She understood Kevin's dilemma and agreed with me that he was suffering from drug-induced psychosis. She understood Kevin's story, his PTSD and drug use, and their interconnectedness. I reassured her that as soon as he was discharged we would work together on a treatment plan.

There were many legal factors that had to be considered. Kevin had previous charges against him as a result of aggressive outbursts, and for this reason, he feared that he would go to prison. Upon his discharge he came back to my office, looking like a scared boy.

I connected with his foster parents; and they supported Kevin by covering his legal fees and so on. During the first few of our weekly sessions, Kevin was again struggling with full-blown trauma. All the symptoms remained active. He had recurrent nightmares about the event on the mountain and his time in prison and the hospital. He was distrustful and felt that the world was against him: He stood alone. No one understood him. He expressed paranoia but was in contact with reality. During many sessions he just sat and wept; he was very sad. He was taking antipsychotic medication and had to check in regularly with a forensic psychiatrist and his probation officer.

This was the most trying time for Kevin. He did not want to give up smoking cannabis; he said that it was his medicine and was helping him. We talked at length about harm reduction and tapering off, but he was reluctant. This was a stormy time for us all.

A few months later he was still deeply depressed, and I encouraged him to connect with his doctor. He resumed his antidepressants, and Hannah walked with him through this painful process. As he came out of the sadness, he began to struggle with rage. Most of his anger was directed at Hannah. On several occasions, he became physical to the point that she had to get a restraining order against him. This devastated Kevin even more.

One day he sat in my office and begged to be released from this internal demon, which he called the darkness. That day he signed his second contract with me to work on his anger and drug use. From then on, things began to look up. He began to embrace his own healing journey. He revisited all the past traumatic experiences in his life. Layer by layer he let go, and the change came. He proposed to Hannah, and they got married. The young couple went through some stormy times as they struggled to find their footing; but they loved each other dearly, and through their love and commitment, they healed.

Kevin's Story in His Own Words

Teresa Marsh helped save my life. She taught me the importance of self-care, to take good care of myself. Before I met Teresa I nearly ended my life on a bridge. Seeing Teresa helped me gain confidence about myself and helped to bring peace to my spirit. I feel that it is important to be truthful with yourself. If someone needs to see someone for therapy, it is important that they seek the therapy. Therapy is as vital as seeing a doctor when you have an injury.

However my injury was depression and PTSD. Teresa helped me repair my soul and gave me the tools to live a better life.

I lost my father when I was twelve years old; he died at a young age, thirty-nine. Losing my father was very tough for me. I had a hard time focusing in school and being happy. I am thankful that Teresa never gave up on me. She would phone me and check in with me to see how I was doing. That is more than what most professionals would do. She always has been positive and kind. She taught me to be kind. She said that when people treat you negatively, don't ever give in to their negativity. She said that negativity is a vicious cycle. She said, "Instead, be positive and know that people don't have the right to treat you in a negative way."

Teresa has so much knowledge and strength. Teresa has the knowledge of spirit. Spirituality is vital in the healing process because spirit is truly who we are. As Teresa and I have discussed on many occasions, people on earth have forgotten their spiritual roots. Some people are stressed out over material things all the time. Time is precious, and we must all work together collectively to bring healing at a global level. I am a new person, connected, grounded, and safe, because of my work with Teresa Marsh.

Conclusion

I am not going to underplay how challenging it was to do this work with Kevin. During the trying times I always remembered what a mentor in South Africa taught me when I was doing psychiatric nursing. She watched me from a distance during a medicine round. I was working in a hospital with the severely mentally ill, and all forty clients in that unit were psychotic, out of contact with reality. They were all heavily sedated, and I was struggling to find the right client to administer the medication to. I was twenty-one years old and so scared I was shaking.

At the end of that medicine round my mentor called me to her office. She said, "Man, you look scared, and that will not help you working with this population. I guess all you can see is the symptoms and the disease. Let me tell you something today, Nurse:

In every sick individual that you see, deep down inside there resides a healthy one. Do not focus on the disease but focus on the healthy human part of your clients. If you can do that, you will be the best psychiatric nurse."

I took it all in, and I changed my attitude that day. I began to look deeply to find that human being, that soul—and it worked! All my fears disappeared, and I became the best psychiatric nurse. I worked in the most challenging areas in psychiatry and thrived with this new attitude. It was amazing. I carried that with me to date. I never give up on any human being. We as humans strive for the same things: healing, peace, and love.

I know Kevin's story is the story of many young people in this world. Healing is a process, and we have to allow and trust the process to unfold gently with all the love and compassion we can find deep within our souls. When we realize our position and the depth of our intimacy with clients and when we begin to appreciate this privilege, we begin to transform. When we are transformed by the acts of giving and caring, we begin to be nourished by these connections. This transformation has taken place in front of my very eyes.

I have witnessed many rewards and much wisdom because of this work. My giving became my receiving. In the giving was sharing; in the sharing was understanding; in the understanding was joy and love and laughter; and I do believe that is what it means to be human.

Kevin now lives in China with his beautiful wife Hannah. I get updates via e-mail from time to time.

Chapter Eight

Violence in Marginalized Communities

Introduction

The Chinese term for *crisis* can be translated "dangerous opportunity." Such an opportunity came to me not long ago; I remember the day so well. Superintendent Keith Forde, who is now deputy chief of police in Toronto, called a meeting to look at a very huge problem in Toronto: violence.

From every corner of Toronto, in areas such as Malvern Scarborough, Lawrence Heights, Jane and Finch, Regent Park, Rexdale, and others, there have been unresolved murders of youth through gun violence. Young, innocent victims were dying daily; these were all unresolved deaths and unexplained violence and murders.

When the time of the meeting came, as I walked into the room, I wondered what would happen that night. I was asking many internal questions, the same questions I had asked when I was in South Africa, during the riots and in the war zones. Many of those questions still remain unanswered.

At that time I was the manager for a SAPACCY program at the Centre for Addiction and Mental Health in Toronto. I was working with high-risk black youth, some severely traumatized, some with addiction to substances, some homeless, some just out of juvenile prison, and so on.

I sat in a room with over twenty-five mothers who were in deep mourning, grieving the deaths of their sons. The room was also filled with police and investigators assigned to those unresolved murders. Sadness filled the room. It was a familiar sadness, one I had experienced many times in South Africa: sadness coupled with helplessness, hopelessness, and a deep painful anger, a sadness that left many unanswered questions.

The dialogue began. The mothers wanted to know why their sons had been killed. They wanted to know if the murderers would be brought to justice. They asked why they could not get answers. They talked about how unsafe the areas they lived in were, the lack of safety in their homes, relationships, and communities, and between men and women, parents and children, and the elderly and their caregivers. They stated that the problem of violence have reached a level of awareness that some called *epidemic*. Crime was one of the top issues in political debates, but there were no answers. Tears came; accusations came; yet there were no answers.

I sensed the pain, grief, and hurt. I stood up and spoke. I took myself back to Cape Town, South Africa, and talked about the 1976 and 1986 riots, when the police opened fire on our children. I told those mothers that at that time we as women did not have a clue as to how much strength, fight, and courage we had left. But it was our children who were being affected. We could not fall into our grief and give up. We had joined together and begun to look at what it was we could do to heal ourselves, those children who were still alive and scared, and the elderly who were so devastated by all of it. We had to look into our hearts to find a way to deal with the trauma, hurt, pain, and uncertainty. We had to find meaning in all the suffering. I told stories about courage, love, faith, and hope. We, the women of Africa, began to focus on what could be done. We started support groups. We met at each other's homes for meals. We told our stories; and we listened; and we began to heal. We began to find new strength and hope as we realized that we were not alone. We changed our attitudes; we became proactive and involved so we could believe and heal. I talked about trauma, loss, grief. and bereavement.

Something shifted profoundly in the energy in that room. I remember that a woman stood up and spoke, who is today my dear friend. Her name is Audette Shephard, and her only son had been brutally shot down and murdered. She spoke with pain in her heart but with determination to do something beyond what was happening in the communities. The rest is history because out of this meeting UMOVE was born: United Mothers Opposing Violence Everywhere!

As we move into the positive and transformative aspect of this story, I need to say a few very important things about trauma, violence, grief, bereavement, and internalized oppression.

Trauma

The task of addressing traumatic experiences and abuse is emerging as one of the most challenging for health care professionals globally. The identification and recognition of trauma and abuse as a major social problem was initiated by the courageous work of the woman's movement or the feminist movement. The people in this movement challenged the inevitability of a patriarchal system that accepts the exploitation of smaller and physically weaker individuals. They explored ways of interrelating through cooperation and mutual respect, rather than seeing violence and competition as the only means of resolving differences (Lew 1990). Judith Herman, MD (Herman 1992) has referred to the need for a movement that ensures that information about trauma doesn't need to be rediscovered every hundred years. Without a movement to remind and reinforce key truths, the best research data are ignored. Society at large (including mental health professionals) finds it less stressful to look the other way instead of dealing with these issues head-on.

Atrocities and trauma involve horrible things that often people don't want to hear about. Bearing witness to horrible events, changes and scars beliefs about the world, one's self, and others. People are traumatized either directly or indirectly, according to the DSM-1V diagnosis of PTSD (APA 1994). They can be traumatized without actually being physically harmed or threatened by harm. Simply learning about traumatic events can carry traumatic potential.

Types of Trauma

Simultaneous trauma: Several members are affected; this can include natural disasters.

Vicarious trauma: Pertains to war, hostage situations, distant disasters, and mine accidents.

Interfamilial trauma or abuse: When one family member causes emotional trauma to another member.

Chasmal or secondary trauma: Traumatic stress that appears to infect the entire system after first appearing in only one member of the group.

Most of the research literature has focused primarily on sexual abuse, with physical abuse being studied to a lesser extent. A few investigators, however, have explored the impact of other kinds of abuse on functioning, including:

- psychological abuse and neglect;
- negative home atmosphere;
- physical neglect;
- emotional withdrawal;
- inconsistency in parenting;
- childhood separations;
- political persecution;
- imprisonment and torture;
- murder; and
- violence.

Traumatic events call into question basic human relationships. Trauma breaches the attachments of families, friendships, love, and community. It shatters the self that is formed and sustained in relation to others. When truth is finally recognized, survivors can begin their recovery.

Grief and Bereavement

Whether dying or bereaved, all people experience grief as a response to death. *Grief* is the affective or emotional response caused by the significant loss of something or someone important to a person. Grief differs in intensity and in the duration of the time needed to resolve the loss. *Bereavement* is the term used to refer to the experiences that follow the death of a loved one, and *mourning* is the term used to describe the social customs and cultural practices that follow a death.

The fears that accompany clients and their families during these times are real; they are normal reactions to an unfavorable diagnosis, crisis, or devastating news. The death of a loved one or facing one's own death can immobilize a person's strengths and increase his or her fears.

Internalized Oppression

External oppression is the unjust exercise of authority and power by one group over another. It includes imposing one group's belief system, values, and life ways over another group. External oppression becomes internalized oppression when someone comes to believe the oppressor's belief system, values, and life way and act as if they are reality. The terms *self-hate* and *internalized racism* are other ways of referring to internalized oppression.

The result of internalized oppression is shame and the disowning of one's own individual and cultural reality. Without internalized oppression, we would not have the previously unseen levels of violence, especially against women and children, that we see today. Internalized oppression means the oppressor doesn't have to exert any more pressure on the oppressed because they exert this pressure on each other and themselves. The divide-and-conquer strategy works. But we resist internalized oppression by learning how to live respectfully and harmoniously together—without violence.

After speaking to over twenty-five mothers who had experienced the loss of a son or daughter, I was convinced that we were dealing with deep intrapsychic trauma and more. I began to walk the streets of Toronto in the areas where violence most often occurred and spoke to as many youth as I could find. I asked them why so many of our youth were dying by the hands of their peers. What came through during these dialogues was that it appeared to the youth, because of the way that they were treated, that they had been assigned this role by society. Because of continuous marginalization, oppression, and racism, they felt dehumanized, devalued, judged, and discriminated against.

It is said that those who are violently oppressed tend to react violently to their oppression. When their violent acts, in their own defense or in reaction to their oppressors, cannot be directed to self-liberation, they are often directed toward each other. The youth told me that, with a weapon such as a gun in their hands, they began to feel powerful beyond measure. Many of the youth had lost faith and hope in themselves and others. They did not trust. Poverty and rejection also played major roles in this. It was clear to me that we needed a powerful message and intervention that could give our youth new strength and hope.

So This Is Trauma ... Now What?

We know as clinicians that dramatization requires both internal and external resources that are inadequate to cope with external threat. We now have a better understanding of what traumatized people are endeavoring to cope with within themselves. It is vital to recognize how difficult or impossible it is for traumatized people to "pull themselves together." They are, in fact, doing it themselves—caught in a recursive loop that informs them that they must continue to fight for their lives, long after the original threat is over. They cannot control how their bodies automatically respond. They cannot command that their memories be properly restored. They are trapped in the tragedy of human existence.

The only real solution to people dealing with this reality is the healing power of others and love. We must understand more about the profound way in which other people determine the ultimate outcome of the traumatic experience. Other people are external resources: our family, friends, neighbors, co-workers, bosses, schoolmates, teachers, administrators, clergymen, and anyone who represents our social group. These external resources can either be the sources of our problems or the sources of our solutions.

It is a fundamental and absolute moral responsibility that we each find a way to bear witness to the pain and suffering that are all around us. Starting from a position of this testimony, we must join together as people to liberate the human body, mind, and spirit from the traumatic reenactment that is stretching our social body, our communities, our people, and our children to the limits of human endurance.

The Courage of a Woman: Audette Shepherd and UMOVE in Her Own Words

I was born in a small town named Princes Town on the beautiful island of

Trinidad and Tobago. I am the fifth of the six surviving children of Elton and Ursula, Constance Shepherd. I had an amazing childhood, free from crime and violence, where we often slept with our doors and windows open through the night. I was considered a tomboy because I loved to climb trees, play boy games, and usually made makeshift boy toys like go-karts and spinning tops. I was also extremely good at track and field.

We were not well-to-do, but we were very happy in our neighborhood. My father was an electrician at the Pointe-a-Pierre oil refinery, and my mom stayed at home to take care of us.

On August 21, 1970, I migrated to Canada and lived with my cousins, hoping to have a better life. I attended school, and upon graduating I secured my first job at the Canadian Imperial Bank of Commerce on March 11, 1974. I started working in the data center and moved through the ranks to become manager of client service, remaining with CIBC until 2002. I am currently employed with Scotia Bank as manager, trade finance and global transactions banking.

Back in 1977, after two previous failed relationships, I started a relationship with a man named Garth. On February 21, 1982, God blessed me with a wonderful baby boy, who I named Justin Garth

Shepherd. Justin was the best thing that ever happened to me. I loved that child more than life itself. As a single mom, I always provided for his needs, and we had a good life. He was the absolute joy of my life; nothing or no one could compare to the love I felt for my son.

God blessed Justin with extraordinary athletic ability. By the time he was in grade eight he was six feet three inches tall and dunking in basketball games and was usually awarded the MVP award. He was considered the most promising basketball prospect in Ontario. By the time he reached grade nine he was considered the best in Canada. In 1983 my relationship with Garth ended. In 1991 I married a man named Magdy. Our marriage ended in 1995. We are still friends, and he recently admitted that he was jealous of the love I had for Justin.

Justin's development became the number one priority in my life. I was always involved with his school and present at all his basketball games and practices. I developed meaningful and maternally nurturing relationships with many of his friends and other youth who would affectionately call me Shep Mom since most of Justin's friends would call him Sheepdog or Shep. Justin's favorite name for me was Mom Dukes.

Donna Langille, who still teaches at Eastern Commerce, was Justin's all-time favorite teacher. He often said that she was the best teacher in the world. I still have a very wonderful relationship with her, and many times we would often reflect on so many funny and endearing memories of Justin.

Justin's dream was to join his half brother Jamaal Magloire in the NBA. This was not any far-fetched hoop dream. Justin had the potential to be a world-class basketball player. When one of Jamaal's friends saw Justin play ball, he remarked that Jamaal better watch it because his little brother would eat his food. Justin had just accepted a scholarship to Maryland and was really excited about it. Unfortunately, tragedy hit on June 23, 2001. Justin was at home when he received a phone call on his cell phone. He said he would be back in ten minutes and left the house, but he never made it back home. He was found shot to death on the Rosedale foot bridge.

When I found out about my son's death, I didn't know what to do with myself. I was overcome with grief. I tried sitting in the couch, but that didn't help. I tried lying in bed but without relief. I started rolling on the floor and screaming but could not find any relief. I didn't want to be me anymore. I couldn't bear the way I felt and wanted to be someone else. The pain was so horrendous. I cried out to God, "But, God, I prayed to you all the time to protect that child, I prayed to you for every mother's son, every mother's daughter. God, how come you couldn't save my child?" God never answered me.

At that time it would have been easy to say, "God, forget you. I don't need you. How could you allow this to happen to me?" I found out that you never really get to know God until he is all you have. I found myself totally dependant on God. I could feel his strength and guidance. He became the God of all comfort, the source of my strength. When people say to me that I am a very strong woman, I say to them, "The joy of the Lord is my strength."

I also found out that out of much sorrow comes much resolve. I developed a very strong passion and commitment to make a difference in our community so that other families do not suffer this horrifying experience. I first started an organization called Brother's Keepers Network along with a local lawyer, Courtney Betty, my pastor, Ainsworth Keith Morris, and former MPP Alvin Curling.

One day I received a call from Superintendent Keith Forde, who is now deputy chief of police in Toronto. He had gathered a number of mothers who lost their children to violence, along with some other police officers, Mike Boyd, Robert Clarke, Jane Wilcox, James Sneep, Nick Memme, Winston LaRoche, Charlene Edwards, Teresa Marsh, and Father Massey Lombardi. Out of this meeting UMOVE was formed. I am currently the Chair of UMOVE (United Mothers Opposing Violence Everywhere).

I also became a director of Toronto Crime Stoppers, resigning in 2006. I was appointed as a board member of the attorney general of Ontario's Office of Victims of Crime. Currently I'm a member of Mayor David Miller's advisory committee for community safety. I also volunteer as a member of the Seventh-Day Adventist prison ministry program at Toronto East Detention Centre.

Justin's death was a life-changing event for me. I have since become a very strong advocate for justice, support for victims of crime, and community safety. I have since received several awards for my efforts, including the Bob Marley Award, the Maja Award for "Woman of Courage," the Scotiabank Global Transaction Banking "Woman of Distinction Award," the African Canadian Achievement Award, and the Scotiabank Global Transaction Banking "Global Citizen Award." Even though my passion comes from within and it's not really about receiving reward or awards, I do appreciate the recognition.

As of this date no one has been arrested for my son's murder. I often think of that night and wonder about his last moments after he was shot. Did he try to call me; did he try to get up; and did he suffer? Some people say that time is the greatest healer, but time has stood still in my heart for the severe pain of the loss of my only child.

If I could have been with Justin 24/7 I would have been there. I couldn't go to bed if he was not at home. I would call him on his cell constantly. I remember once he said to me, "Mom, you are a stalker. Stop stalking me." Another time he said, "Don't worry, Mom. Everything is crisp. Everything is gravy." But it wasn't crisp and it wasn't gravy that night when they ended my son's life, ended his dreams, my dreams, and the dreams of an entire community. So many people knew about Justin's athletic ability and were looking forward to seeing him join his brother in the NBA. Every mother knows that when you give birth to a child, every part of you, everything you eat, think, or feel, becomes an integral part of that child. When Justin died, a huge part of me died with him.

I am a member of the prayer group at my church, and I would often pray a very angry prayer. "God, you know who killed Justin. Give them no rest and no peace. Go find them and bring them to justice." One Sabbath a very dear old man who I cared for deeply, Brother William Peart, who is now deceased, said to me, "Sister Shephard, you cannot go to God with all that anger and bitterness in your heart. You have to let go and let God." I did not respond to him, but on my drive home, I was crying and so angry with him because I felt he did not have the right to tell me anything as he had not lost his son.

My entire afternoon was a total wreck. That night I got on my knees and cried out to God and asked him to take charge because I couldn't do it on my own. I started to pray and found myself giving God thanks for the nineteen years he gave me Justin, for all the love, the happiness, and the companionship that Justin brought into my life. I thanked God for his promise that vengeance belongs to him and he will repay. I asked God to help me not to be so obsessed with vengeance.

When I finished that prayer I felt something physically lifted from my chest. At that moment I decided that my expectations were from God. It was no longer from the police or people who had information that they would not come forward with. I believed in my heart that there would be justice for Justin, so I no longer roamed the streets seeking information. Some days though, I still get consumed with seeking vengeance myself because I feel like I owe it to Justin to find his murderer and make him pay. But then I say a prayer and ask God to keep my mind on him and to keep me in perfect peace. I can honestly tell you that sometimes the quest for justice and closure can suck the very life of out of you.

At the moment of Justin's death, witnesses reported three people running from the scene. Strangely enough, I was looking out my window and also saw the three people running, and they entered into a side door of an apartment building. I did not make much of it at the time but later found out whom they were. I spoke to one of their mothers, and she said she would ensure that her son would speak to the police. I gave her the detective's number so her son could call. The next day a lawyer phoned the detective and advised that his client was not interested in speaking with him.

It broke my heart; I couldn't understand how a nineteen year old could be a client in this situation. As painful as it was, I realized that there are no winners in this situation; there is one mother who lost her only son and another mother who is worried about losing her son to jail.

I thank God for the relationship I have with him because if I didn't have the love of God in my heart I would probably be in jail or dead at this time, due to the temptation to get hold of a gun and shoot everyone who I felt had information or was a part of the situation.

There is not one day that I do not think of Justin, of what could have been, of his beautiful smile, his humor, of that child who to me was the best son in the world. I remember when he was sixteen years old and he kept begging me for a tattoo on his arm. I told him I did not like the idea. He begged constantly until I finally gave in. When he turned eighteen, he told me he was getting another one. I told him not to do so. Two months before his death I came home from work and noticed something just under his T-shirt.

"Jus, you got a tattoo?" I asked.

"Nah, man," he said and pulled away.

When I saw the tattoo, I was speechless.

"Yeah, Mom ... What?" He had my name tattooed onto his chest. I said to him, "But, Jus, how come my name? I thought you would put a girl's name." There were so many girls that were interested in him.

He said, "Mom, a girl? Let me tell you this, Mom, there is no one in this world that I love more than you." He slapped his hand on his chest and said, "I will tell you that right now."

I will cherish that moment for the rest of my life. The Bible says that there is no greater love than when a man would lay down his life for a friend. I cannot promise that I would lay my life down for a friend, but I would certainly have laid it down for my son.

I continue living day by day trying to empower youth to make the right choices in life and to climb the staircase of life one step at a time, because life is not about "bling bling." We have all been blessed with unique gifts, and we should utilize our gifts to our full potential. Never be jealous of someone's gift because you have your own.

Doing my community work has become a tremendous catharsis for me and keeps Justin's legacy alive in my heart. There are times when I get a bit discouraged, when members of UMOVE don't step up to the plate or demonstrate the commitment I expect from them. I always remember that it's not about me. It's about every mother's son and every mother's daughter that I can make a difference for. I will continue to do whatever I can to promote peace, love, safety, and preservation of life for all communities.

My call to action came when my son was murdered; I implore everyone to let your call to action be now. Don't wait for tragedy to hit before you get involved with your community's safety. Mahatma Gandhi once said, "You never know what results can come from your action, but if you do nothing, there can be no results." Crime anywhere is a threat to safety everywhere.

Shortly after Justin was murdered, I met Teresa at the meeting called by Superintendent Keith Ford to address the recent state of violence in Toronto. Teresa had not lost a child, but she attended as a means of support for the mothers. When we were introduced to each other, there was an instant spiritual connection. She seemed wise beyond her years. She was a strong sense of support and resiliency to me and the other mothers. I remember when the trauma of loss created moments of conflict among the mothers, Teresa always created a stabilizing force to bring structure and resolution. A few years ago Teresa moved to Vancouver, and our spiritual connection continues to bind us together in a very meaningful friendship. Thank you, my friend, for including me in your book and giving me an opportunity to tell my story once again.

Conclusion

No matter who we are, we are always driven by an internal energy in the search for complete wholeness and peace. Each step that we take on life's long journey brings us closer to that place of being. We may appear to step away from our divine paths, yet all steps eventually lead us forward. Even the most horrific and tragic happenings and losses can lead to new ways of being and grace. It is in the darkness that light shines the brightest. When things get really low and we get totally disillusioned with life and the material gains it offers, we search for something more. We want to know the reason for our pain and suffering. When in the depths of suffering, we are forced to look at that wounded place with our eyes open. When we do, we find that internal light, that strength and hope and peace—in other words, that spirit within. When we look within, we find the bliss of the divine.

Illness, the death of a loved one, fear, pain, and suffering can all introduce us to an inner peace that we never knew before; they deliver the message of what life is really about. Life is a one-way journey toward our divine selves. All ups and downs are just stops along the way where we learn more of life's lessons to move forward.

Chapter Nine

Altered Body Image

Introduction

Any visible or invisible disfigurement of the body can have a profound psychological effect on a person. It can impinge on one's quality of life, self-esteem, and social encounters; thus the psychosocial implications can be horrific. The effects can infiltrate a person's entire being in the physical, emotional, social, cultural, and spiritual dimensions.

This chapter follows Jade's story. Jade was diagnosed with polycystic ovarian syndrome at age eighteen, but in her case, the trauma occurred long before the diagnosis because she was misdiagnosed. Her suffering began as soon as she entered puberty when she was confronted with a host of changes in her body.

First Visit

Jade was referred to me by her mother, who was very worried about the unhappiness and fear that her daughter had been living with for so many years. Even though she was a university student by then, she was still very unhappy and needed some healing and help.

Jade presented at my office a year ago when she was twenty-three; she was an attractive, slim, and tall brunette, who was very shy and withdrawn. She stated that she had come for therapy because she had been plagued for so many years by body image and self-esteem issues, loneliness, singlehood, depression, anxiety, and excessive worry. She had felt isolated for most of her life, and the biggest pain was that she felt different. She felt like an outcast or, as she later put it, a "freak." Unlike the other students at her school, who were dating and having a good time, she was isolated and avoided dating and enjoying her life. She had been on antidepressants since the age of sixteen years, but she wanted to live without the help of medication.

At age sixteen she was referred to a counselor, but at that time she was so ashamed and disgusted by her condition that she could not bring herself to talk about her problems. After high school she attempted therapy again and managed to stick with it for six months. She said that it had helped her somewhat. She then moved to Toronto to complete a course in jewelry design technology. After a year she came back to Vancouver and studied at Langara College. When she came to see me, she was completing an art history degree.

Altered Body Image and Trauma

Jade stated that she had always been self-conscious about her body—even as early as the age of six. She was shy and felt awkward in her body. She used to play with Barbie dolls and watched all the stories on television about beauty, love, beautiful princesses, and how only beautiful girls got the princes. This impacted her deeply, and she began to view these stories as truth. She had a very loving and kind mother who always told her that she was beautiful, but Jade felt that she had already been influenced by the media even at such a young age. All her friends had Barbies and had the same ideas about women and beauty.

Puberty usually occurs between the ages ten and fourteen. During this time the body produces extra amounts of chemicals called hormones that cause the body to undergo physical and emotional changes, including increased height, changes in body shape, the growth of breasts and pubic hair, and so on. This period is also coupled with mood swings that come and go.

This was when the trouble started for Jade because all of her friends were changing and talked openly about the changes. Jade was changing as well—but in a different way. She started to grow hair all over her body, legs, and arms. She remained flat-chested, and unlike the other girls, her period did not come. She was devastated by this and began to feel shame about her body. Brutal and negative thoughts began to plague her mind, telling her that she was a freak, that she was being punished for something she had done, and that no one would ever want to be with her. She started to cover herself up, wearing long sleeves in hot weather and so on. Also, because she was carrying this secret, she began to isolate herself. She became very sad, and at times felt that she just wanted to die. She suffered on her own.

Traumatic Event

One day she was changing in the washroom after a physical education class. She always made sure that she stood in a far corner when she changed, but on this day, one of her friends came by and saw the hair on her chest and arms. The friend did not say anything to her but informed the other girls in their group. These friends then sent one of the girls to ask Jade to lift up her sweater. Jade then realized that the word was out, and of course she was devastated and also alienated from her group. The result was more isolation, fear, guilt, shame, pain, and suffering.

By this time, she was thirteen, and finding it unbearable to carry on on her own, she confided in her mother. Her mother was very supportive, agreed about the abnormality, and took Jade to see the doctor. At the doctor's office Jade was told that her condition was nothing to be concerned about but was normal for some young girls. The doctor also added that it could be related to the fact that she was of Eastern European decent. This traumatized her even more and she began to question why, if this was all normal, she had such horrible feelings about it. Why was she so sad, and why did she feel from time to time that she wanted to die? Again, the harsh ego voice told Jade that she was a freak.

Jade's mom was her main support and encouraged and reassured her. She had two siblings, an older and a younger brother, who were both very smart—far smarter than she was, she often said. They were loving and kind and so was her father. With their love and support, Jade could tolerate her condition better. But the ego mind grew stronger as she tried to minimize her feelings. She was depressed and having suicidal thoughts. Her emotional state affected her functioning at school, and she struggled with her grades.

Polycystic Ovary Syndrome

Polycystic ovary syndrome (PCOS) is an endocrine disorder that affects approximately 5 percent of all women. (Tan, Hahn, Benson, et al 2007). It occurs amongst all races and nationalities and is the most common hormonal disorder of women of reproductive age as well as a leading cause of infertility. The principle features are obesity, anovulation (resulting in irregular menstruation), acne, and excessive amounts or effects of androgenic (masculinizing) hormones. Other symptoms include hirsutism (excessive and increased body hair, typically in a male pattern, affecting the face, chest, and legs), depression, deepening of the voice, and weight gain.

At that time Jade's most debilitating symptoms were excessive hair, irregular periods, and depression. She had only slight weight gain, as she was always very conscious of maintaining her weight. She had not yet been diagnosed, even though she went for second opinions. She was started on anti-depressants at age sixteen.

During the last three years of high school, while others were having fun and enjoying life, Jade became more isolated and sad. She watched television shows that confronted her more and more with the worldview of women that indicated true beauty amounted to being slim and pretty. She came to believe she was an outcast and a freak. She suffered at a very deep level, and the trauma that surrounded all of this became more and more invasive. By the time she walked into a counselor's office, she was so damaged that she did not feel she deserved to be listened to. She had given up.

Her mother intervened in her supportive way and encouraged

Jade to go for laser hair removal. During this time, Jade's anxiety was also inspired by the fact that she felt she had the most horrible-looking nose. She shared this with her mother, and her mother reassured her that, if she wanted, she could have plastic surgery. She described the anxiety this way: "I hated my nose. I hated my body."

Jade started the laser therapy at age seventeen, and it was both traumatic and therapeutic. It was traumatic to expose her body to a stranger because it was so shameful to her. Jade's anxiety was heightened at this time, and she suffered at a very deep level.

The Diagnosis

Jade was finally diagnosed when she was nineteen. Jade's mom was talking to a family member and friend about Jade's sadness and condition. This friend knew a family member with the same issues and told Jade's mom that it had a name, a diagnosis, and could be treated! Back to the doctor they went, and Jade's mom told the doctor about her conversation with her friend. Finally Jade was properly examined and diagnosed.

The diagnosis was a revelation; now Jade's suffering had a name, and proper treatment could be implemented. Jade's doctors discovered the cysts on her ovaries, which fortunately could be dealt with. I think that the greatest relief for Jade was that she was validated about all the things she had felt were not right. This was when things began to shift for Jade. Three years later she accepted therapy and healing into her life. As time went by she came to realize that she mattered and that she was indeed beautiful. She did not reflect what was dictated about beauty in the media; she was beautiful in her own right.

Beauty and Body Image in the Media

The American research group Anorexia Nervosa and Related Eating Disorders reports that one out of every four college-aged women uses unhealthy methods of weight control, including fasting, skipping meals, excessive exercise, laxative abuse, and self-induced vomiting. The pressure to be thin is affecting young girls. In Jade's situation, her weight was not a major issue, but needless to say, she struggled all the same. The images of females are everywhere, and Jade was exposed to this from a very young age. She viewed popular film and television actresses who were taller, thinner, and considered more beautiful. In addition, Jade saw youth, along with thinness, promoted as an essential criterion of beauty. Media images of female beauty are unattainable for all but a very small number of women. But Jade was constantly fed these lies, and due to her poor self-image, these lies were easily enforced. It is no wonder she walked around feeling anxious and half human for most of her young adult life.

Therapy/Healing

After several therapy sessions, Jade slowly came out of her shyness, and I noticed a change in her mood. She was a bit more pleasant and began to trust me. She shared a deeper level of her suffering. She was constantly anxious and fearful. She went through agony and hell, as she completed assignments, papers, and exams. The ego mind would plague her at all levels, and she would go through phases of self-loathing, self-hate, self-deprivation, and punishment. This was her life constantly. This suffering was the norm for her.

During one session I asked Jade the million-dollar question: "So, Jade, what do you want?" Here is the answer she gave me:

- I want to live to my fullest potential and do special things in life.
- I want to connect with my special gifts.
- I want to feel good about myself.
- I want to feel more secure in who I am.
- I want to say yes to opportunities.
- I want to travel.
- I want to date and have a family.
- I want to enjoy life and connect with others.

She finished by telling me that she believed it was all possible. And away we went. In the present Jade believed in herself. Even though she could not totally see how the trauma pain, and suffering had been taken on by her ego as her true self, she had a foundation. I told Jade we could work on the basics. We could do the trauma and healing work, but during all the sessions we were going to work on grounding her in the here and now, helping her to watch her mind in action, and beginning cognitive behavioral therapy to help her work on her self-defeating behaviors. She was validated and supported. I reassured Jade over and over that she could heal from all of these traumatic events. She was ready and happy.

I gave her homework: daily journaling, meditation, thought tracking, safety, and self-care. She could not beat herself up anymore. In the office we started off the sessions with deep breathing, meditation, and visualization. Jade was encouraged to attend yoga classes; she did and loved it. She went back to the gym and began regular workouts. Her mood improved, and she became more open and trusting and continued to tell her story. She began to realize that her story of hurt, pain, and suffering had to be told; as she did, she learned more and more about how her condition and the way it had been handled had affected her. She learned very quickly that it was not her fault; she was not a freak, nor was she just her disease, her thoughts, or her mental formations. She was far more than that. She began to connect more and more with her true self; she began to realize that truth was her identity. She made new friends and started to date. This was all new for her, and she struggled with her self-esteem issues and insecurities. But his did not stop her. She was being cheered on. She went through her first heartbreak and worked through it. She was healing. It was palpable and visible.

Why Yoga?

Yoga means "to unite" mind, body, and spirit. I believed that with yoga exercises Jade would connect with the essence of her mind, body, and spirit—her core self, her true identity, her greatness, and her roots. In yoga we find that place of stillness where we can pause and change the mind, thus we can make informed and healthy decisions about health, wellness, and ourselves and can impact what we think about all day long.

Studies have shown these results in people who practice yoga:

1. Decrease in anxiety, depression, defensiveness, guilt, tension, hostility, and anger.
2. Increase in openness to experience, conflict resolution, self-concept, body image, interpersonal relationships, self-esteem, and ethical self- and spiritual orientation.

It was our hope that the practice of yoga would help Jade deal with the issues and challenges that she faced on a daily basis. By practicing yoga, Jade became more aware of her inner and outer beauty and strengths, and she began to see her own greatness as a young woman.

Why Meditation?

We are always engaged in four different levels of thinking:

1. *Negative thought:* anger, fear, sadness, regret, unease (lowest level)
2. *Wasteful thought:* worrying about things outside of our control
3. *Necessary thought:* concerning things that we have to do, reminders (e.g., grocery lists or bills to pay)
4. *Positive thought:* highest form of thought, which encourages peace, harmony, creativity, love, and happiness

Because of the trauma Jade experienced, she mainly stayed engaged in levels one, two, and three. In meditation we can free our minds from negative and wasteful thoughts and elevate them to the highest level. That is exactly what the meditation started doing for Jade. She learned fast about the mind, ego mind, and higher self.

Practicing yoga and meditation are powerful, transforming, healing, and revealing! I highly recommend this to all my clients. I have witnessed profound results, even after just one session. In all of us resides the most powerful part of our being, the true self, the higher self, the soul, the spirit, our essence; there are many names for it. This part of us can only be accessed when we are quiet, still, and paying attention. Therefore meditation is what I call the medicine, the elixir, and the *muti* that lead us into that realm. As we cultivate a practice, profound things emerge at a very subtle level and these include:

- Stress relief;
- Relaxation;
- Better concentration;
- Increased self-awareness;
- A clear sense of purpose;
- A sense of well-being; and
- A Positive attitude about life.

Meditation changed my life. It made me realize that the ego mind, the constantly chattering mind, is dangerous, mean, cruel, nasty, and hateful and lives only in the past or the future. I realized that it had no space or place when I lived in the present—the here and now. I realized that, if I was not aware, the ego could rob me of all the beautiful things in life. I share this with all clients.

Jade's Story in Her Own Words

Looking back on my life, it is hard to remember a time that I didn't feel uncomfortable within my own skin. From a very early age I remember feeling uncomfortable in bathing suits and any form-fitting clothing. Although I was slim child I was always conscious of how I appeared to others and did my best to avoid being too exposed. I remember spending countless hours as I grew up looking in the mirror and wondering how I stacked up, whether I was beautiful or attractive enough. I saw attractive women in my favorite TV shows, on pageants, or the cheerleaders at the nearby high school, and in my young developing mind, I equated physical beauty with greatness, popularity, and social acceptance. While those thoughts were diluted, they did not cause a great hindrance to my self-concept until about grade seven when I began to go through puberty. It was during this awkward time of transition that I noticed a large change in my body that alarmed me. I began to see the appearance of fine black hair, which appeared on my stomach, back, and chest. When I looked in the mirror I was devastated, as I did not see beauty but deformity and all the makings of what I considered a freak.

For over a year after the excessive hair appeared, I lived with my secret. To me there was so much shame, so much disgust for my own body, that I couldn't bear to let anyone else know my truth. I covered my body and avoided any situation in which it might be exposed, which at times proved challenging. Because of my shame, I also avoided boys and the dating scene, which only made me feel further alienated from my peers who were getting those experiences. The problem seemed so large, so unmanageable, I was overwhelmed, depressed, and self-loathing. Although I never planned out a suicide, it remained in my mind as a way one day to escape what I thought was an unbearable future trapped within my body.

After a time I finally found the courage to tell my mom, who became a great source of support in my journey. The years that followed were comprised of numerous doctor visits in order to understand what was causing the hair growth. These doctor visits all came back with disheartening results, some claiming there was nothing biologically wrong, others attributing it to genetics. The fact that I was unable to get a diagnosis only seemed to reinforce my fears that there truly was something innately wrong with me and with my body.

At age eighteen I was finally diagnosed with polycystic ovarian syndrome thanks to the suggestion of a family friend whose daughter had been recently diagnosed. Being diagnosed with polycystic ovarian syndrome brought a number of positive changes into my life as I began to understand I was not a freak or alone in my struggle. Although there is no cure for PCOS I have been on a number of medications to regulate my hormones and the side effects, and over the years have been fortunate to have laser therapy sessions for the reduction of my hair growth. The laser hair removal has been a form of therapy in itself, allowing me to shed myself of the hair and its underlying pain. These changes have allowed me to see my body in new ways and begin to see my problems as manageable.

Although the physical changes that were happening to my body were great, there still remained a powerful ego mind within me that was insecure and scarred from the pain of my past. These issues were holding me back from life experiences such as dating, which at age twenty-three I had not experienced.

Seeking help to heal my past wounds, I encountered Teresa through a recommendation on my mom's behalf. She was a student in one of Teresa's yoga class and had come home raving about her excellent teacher. When she learned that Teresa offered counseling services, she was quick to grab her card and encouraged me to call as soon as I could.

Walking into Teresa's office for the first time I felt I had entered the right space, as it was unlike the typical stark psychotherapy offices I had visited prior but instead held candles and a diverse range of spiritual books and artifacts. I quickly came to learn Teresa's approach to therapy was equally refreshing, as she saw healing as a process that involved mind, body, and spirit.

The initial sessions with Teresa were particularly important in that they allowed me to share a painful part of my being which I had so rarely talked about to anyone. These sessions helped me to understand the transformative power in sharing one's story. After years of living in silence with my inner demons, it allowed me to separate myself from that internal voice and verbalize the emotions I had been feeling all those years. Sharing what has been a difficult and painful aspect of my life has allowed me to see the excessive hair, not as something definitive of me, but as something that *happened* to me.

Teresa's focus on the mind, ego, and spirit in her therapy has been of great benefit to me in my healing process. Most particularly, her emphasis on the ego mind has encouraged me to become more conscious of my thoughts and more accountable to them. Although I can't control the media, or whether I fit the current mold of beauty, I can control how I perceive myself. The meditations that begin each therapy session have encouraged me to develop a stronger relationship with my spirit. It has given me strength but above all a sense of compassion for and self-acceptance of who I am as a person. Feeling a presence of divinity within me has helped me to understand I am not my body but something much greater and eternal.

In the months that followed our first meeting, Teresa introduced me to yoga as a powerful stress reliever and therapeutic aide. I immediately loved the relaxation benefits, but more importantly the new awareness and connection it encouraged me to feel with my own body. Yoga was important in making me, as someone who had body image issues, feel connected to and grateful for the body I have.

Now years after my diagnosis and years of therapy, I feel a different approach to my body that for many years I didn't think was possible. My therapy, with the guidance of Teresa, has ignited me to see my body and spirit in new ways and has given me tools to heal the past and move forward in the future. What at the age of fifteen seemed like a future of pain and shame ahead of me, I now look back at as life lessons, and a testament to my perseverance, strength, and self-love. I have learnt that the large crises we face in life, which to me appeared in the form of hair, are really just journeys that provide opportunities for growth and compassion for others that suffer similarly. I now know that no issue is unmanageable if we approach it day by day, doctor by doctor, or in my case hair by hair.

Conclusion

Jade's story is a sad story with a happy ending. So many women can relate to the pain and suffering in this story. We are each the reflection of the other. We are all connected. I believe that in every clinician, therapist, or healer also lives a wounded one. In every client, every suffering human being, resides a very powerful inner healing. I witnessed this once again on my journey with Jade.

What did it take? Encouragement and support helped Jade to take that journey within, and there she found her own inner healer. There she discovered that truth was her identity. In that discovery she learned to care for herself and to be alive in her living—without judgment and the cruelty of the ego mind. Through the telling of her story, mindfulness meditation, yoga, grounding, focusing, and watching the mind in action, she began to reconnect with her own core and inner strength. Finding that inner strength helped to heal all those old ugly wounds of her past. She began to honor her own truth.

Jade learned that watching the mind in action was her highest form of meditation. She began to think many good things about herself; she moved into the light. In this formula she found her own tranquility, fearlessness, and freedom—in other words, her own inner peace.

Chapter Ten

Healing Is Revealing

Introduction

I believe in the concept of reciprocity in healing sessions. Gifts and surprises come when we are ready or when we least expect them.

Jade and I were about to start a session. She was dealing with her first breakup. She was sad; she talked about the pain in her heart, her anger, bargaining, and the active ego mind that had been so brutal and cruel to her for many years. I listened, supported, held, and reflected. I love story telling during healing sessions. I believe that a story captures the entire universal energy and essence as well as experiences people can relate to.

This young lady loved my stories. I said to her, "You are grieving right now, and that is good. Grieving is a natural part of life and losses. It is good for your soul. Allow your heart to break. Allow your tears to flow; it is so healing. When your heart grows back it will be bigger and stronger." She captured and received the healing words.

"Let me read to you from my little grieving book right here," I continued. "Remember that you are still alive and that is how it should be. Know that your pain has passed, except that now it lives in your memory. You are the one in pain now. It is best to lovingly care for your wounds. You may be disorientated, depressed, and forgetful. These things are normal with grief and will pass. Denying sadness denies grief. By letting your heart break, you let your heart heal. You may experience anger and rage, and you may want to blame someone. Find help to understand and handle your feelings."

As I read, I felt something so profound touching my soul and hers. The energy in the room changed to softness, gentleness, and peace. In this moment descended the gift of wisdom. I said, "Young lady with a broken heart, you just gave me the greatest gift on earth."

She asked, "What is that?"

"An a-ha," I said.

She asked, "An a-ha like in *Oprah*?"

"An a-ha, a moment of wisdom, of knowing. Yes, like in *Oprah*. I am going to write about this, just like in this little grief book, because these moments of sharing such powerfully written words can be profound and priceless. I felt your energy and mine shift the moment I uttered those healing words. I felt it right here in the heart of the matter. Did you feel it?"

"Yes, I did."

"I can now complete that book. I received the title *Enlightenment Is Letting Go*."

"Wow," she said, her eyes smiling. "That is so great."

"See how the universe teaches us. In the mist of your pain you still have these beautiful gifts to offer. I am going to write about your story. Your story will inspire so many young, brokenhearted university students."

"How?" she asked.

"Through poetry, through story telling, through all the wisdom and teachings that I have learned and received from the people I have been working with over the years as a healer and psychotherapist.

"See, the reason why I could not complete the book yet was because I wanted to write about trauma, addiction, loss, grief, bereavement, affliction, hurt, and pain—but not in a negative context. I wanted to approach it in this way, the way it just happened for you. I wanted to capture how people heal, how people in the depth of deep pain and suffering find meaning in the deeper parts of their beings. Your story and experiences can be an elixir and balm for others.

"I saw your transformation and healing here—right here—as I was reading from the little grief book, right?"

"Yes, the words were so powerful. I could feel it."

"Let me tell you the story of the client who was in just before you. He was so sad today, just like you. He was so hurt, just like you. He said that he was 'stuck,' just like you thought you were a few sessions ago. I listened to all his negative comments: 'I can't get it. I am so stuck. I can't get the meditation. I am so dumb. I am so lost. I am so hurt.' Familiar, right?"

She chuckled. "Right, that was me."

"Do you know what I told him? I told him, 'Of course you are all of that, because you say it over and over, and by now you believe that about yourself. If the law of attraction is correct, then your outcomes are bang on!'"

Then I told him a story. As I started to tell the story, he sat back, just as you are sitting right now, ready to listen. Everything changed during the telling of that story. It was not a big change like in your case, but it was a moment of receiving, accepting, and connecting to the other person in the story, the struggles, hurt, and pain. Suddenly he could relate; he felt and realized that he was not alone, struggling in the world all by himself. There were others who felt stuck but became unstuck because they believed in themselves. They took risks; tried new things; and it worked."

Jade smiled a gentle, knowing, soft, curious smile. "Please tell me the story. I want to know."

Our time was almost up, and Jade said that she felt renewed strength and hope; she moved out of her sorrow that day and gave a gift of wisdom. I made my promise to her. I said, "I will write that book for you, and you will read the healing story."

The Healing Story

This story has already healed so many. It is a story about the most brutal ego mind, about betrayal of the self by the self. It is about suffering and healing. It is about the courage of a man and a woman. It is about the revelation of the healing power of love, faith, and hope. As you read the poems in this story, I know that they will touch you in a very deep place within.

At a meeting in my office in Toronto, a client of mine was very upset and concerned about her friend.

"Teresa, I would like you to see this friend of mine. He is a great guy, a good man; he is such a good friend. He needs your help."

I told my client that I was not taking on any new clients, but she pleaded, "He is not an addict, Teresa. He is a good man. He started to have these panic attacks and cannot leave his apartment; he is stuck there."

"You mean I have to go to his apartment?" I asked. By the end of the session, she had convinced me to see her friend.

These two poems tell the story of our first meeting in his apartment building.

Myself Betrayed Me

I am laden with fear, I have come undone
My confidence, my strength, happiness all gone
A few months ago I was on top of the world
Today I am scared to leave the apartment, I feel so old

I feel confused, trapped; mostly scared I'd say
One day I woke up and there was the change to this day
Oh I am so embarrassed, you must think that I am mad
But I'm in a panic and so very sad

I am a writer, film director, successful I think
Now I sense a nervous breakdown on the brink
I struggle to understand the reasons for my state
Things were good, now I loathe self, this condition I hate

A few weeks ago I received news that my script was a great success
The result, I can now create, write and get paid to think and rest
Suddenly I had so many choices, they were just all there
In spite of this good news, this gift, I feel so bare

A beautiful angel entered my life at the same time of the news
She chose to care for me, be with me, now I am even more confused
I could not accept all of this and started to fear all kinds of things
Why is it that I can't accept these beautiful gifts that life brings?

Is it because I have been isolated for so long
Please tell me where have I gone wrong
This state, turmoil is driving me insane, I beg of you?
Can you help someone in my state, what is it that I need to do?

Looking back I realize that I have experienced pains before
I have been through suffering, loneliness many times I just closed the
door
I am kind of shy, quiet, very private and sometimes not so sure
One thing I know, my intentions are always pure

I look, anticipate, waiting for the other shoe to drop
My mind is burdened with horrible fears, I want it to stop
Why now, why here, where did I go wrong?
I feel like a failure, I am weak not strong

What? You ask how I feel about all of this?
I have been talking for one hour, what have you missed?
Hell, now look what is happening to me …
Suddenly I am so sad, I am now crying … please let me be
This is so embarrassing, I really feel so bad
To tell you the truth, all my life I was really very sad

Crisis Call Answered

How do you feel meeting in your space?
You say you do not mind you feel safe in your own place
I sense that there is a lot going on for you right now
Go ahead, I am all ears, tell your story, there is no how

It has been only a few months ago
You received good news, yet you feel so low?
Your burden is great, your suffering profound
You are confused, with anxiety and fear you are hounded

You spoke to so many about your fear and feelings
You were given all good advice and new leads
What you really need is understanding and relief
These gifts are making you feel like a thief?

You feel you are betrayed by your body, spirit and mind?
Your experiences so real, confusing you feel so blind
You cannot understand what has really happened to you?
You say that you have always been kind and true?

Your pain and suffering is great I can tell
It sounds like the past weeks have been a hell
I sense that you really feel confused and lost
Your agony, fear and chaos is not without a cost

I work and approach treatment holistically
My commitment deep, my philosophy truth and reality
I can work with you if you are prepared to do the work
Yes, you can be healed; you are already on the path

In therapy what you do is you borrow a second set of eyes
To help you look deeply into your soul's cries
Healing is possible with work, love and action yes
In the final analysis joy will come, coupled with bliss

Comments

After I met with him for three sessions in his apartment and I set him up with a psychiatrist for collaboration and medication, he came to my office for the first time. He had developed the courage to leave his apartment, and the healing work continued.

Rob was traumatized as a four year old. At the age of four he was taken to the hospital for emergency surgery. He was left there on his own, and his memories of that time were that he was petrified and kept on looking to see if he could spot his mother. But she had left the hospital; she was gone.

As a teenager he was isolated and spent a lot of time on his own, reading and writing. He was always dysthymic. Dysthymia is a type of low-grade depression. The Greek word *dysthymia* means "bad state of mind" or "ill humor." It has fewer and less serious symptoms than major depression but lasts longer. Most dysthymic people cannot tell for sure when they first became depressed.

Traumatic events destroy the sustaining bonds between an individual and others as well as his or her view of self, others, and the world. In the process of trauma a person loses his or her human connections and sense of community. Traumatized individuals often express or display that their sense of self-worth, of humanity, depends upon feelings of connection to others. As Rob and I moved deeper I believed that the energy and healing work could provide the strongest protection against terror and despair and the strongest antidote to further traumatic experiences for Rob.

Rob was petrified and haunted by the stories in his mind. He was plagued by obsessive thoughts that would come and frighten the hell out of him. Then one day he had a full-blown panic attack.

The Attack

Rob was driving to his mother's home one day to pay his parents a visit. As he approached the house, he began to have obsessive thoughts: "You are going to kill your mother." The result was a huge panic attack. He had to stop driving and finally turned back. He was devastated and laden with fear and panic.

Comments

The language that we develop later in life, the language of deep inconsolable pain in Rob's case, is caused by trauma. The language is the symptoms and behaviors we begin to exhibit as the soul goes into hiding at the time of the traumatic event to protect the self. The language spoken is shown through the symptoms, whether depression, anxiety, panic attacks, eating disorders, addiction, or other disorders. Whatever the expression, the turning onto self is initially always about protecting the vulnerable self. We call this coping or defense mechanisms. Later on it becomes pathological, and it begins to hurt the self. We begin to treat ourselves the way we were treated as children.

In therapy, the teaching and education about the mind, body, and spirit are so crucial as a part of the healing journey. We want to know why—why we repeat the same behaviors over and over again when they only produce the same results and outcomes. Alcoholics Anonymous calls that insanity!

The Ego Mind

Rob's symptoms started just as he entered an intimate relationship. Relationships are the foundational grounds between the ego mind and the spirit or true self. Relationships develop in the womb. Each of us is born innocent and pure, with a clean slate and an open heart. We enter the world and become exposed to the fear of parents and the dangers in the world, and then we change to adapt. We are trained to be fearful and untrusting. We get beaten, verbally abused, blamed, and we are made to feel guilt and shame.

The ego takes all of this fear, abuse, blame, and negativity on as truth. As the late B. K. S. Iyengar, one of my spiritual teachers, wrote in his book *Light on Life*, the surface of the ego is covered with superglue, and attached to the superglue is all that ego accumulated. The hurt, pain, wounds, and ego begin to tell us that all of that is who we are. He further states that if we identify with that false value or the ego mind, we place ourselves in unbearable tension. As we identify with this ego, we shut down the higher or true self.

So in Rob's case we had a lot of work to do. In traditional psychotherapy the focus is on personality, weakness, and how to solve it, particularly through identifying what childhood experiences led to the problems. Working as a spiritual healer and psychotherapist, I focus on the experiences and the solutions and then wait for the divine answer.

During our sessions, as Rob continued to lament about this brutal ego mind and its harsh voice, I told him to give it a name and to speak back to the voice with power. When we name something, we gain power over it. I encouraged Rob to take back his power by naming the voice. As Rob began to understand the vicious ego mind and as he began to watch his mind in action, things began to change. One day he told me he had found a name for that harsh ego voice. He was excited as he proclaimed, "And it works!" He had named the voice the Freak Show!

He said, "I was sitting at Starbucks, writing. I looked up and saw a very attractive young man. Then my thoughts, voice, or ego mind said, 'See? You are gay!' The panic feeling was approaching fast. Then I said to the voice, 'Wow, the Freak Show is back. Hello there, Freak Show. You are here again to freak me out. Oh no, you can't do that now. I know who you are, and I am in charge. I am doing the work, and I am changing."

And he was fine—no panic attack. This was a huge shift and change in Rob. He found his footing and his ground; he found his truth. The meditation, support, and healing were working. From there on, things were looking up for Rob.

Comments

For some it takes a long time to understand or to unlearn those old patterns of behavior. In Rob's case he learned very fast; all the interventions in therapy and the healing journey added up. The new skills and learning Rob was exposed to helped tremendously; these included: engaging in meditation, pursuing safety and self-care, watching the mind in action, understanding consciousness, practicing yoga, going for walks and running, eating a healthy diet, drinking lots of water, cutting down on alcohol, reconnecting with family and friends, and finding a new love. Rob found love indeed. I also worked with Shelly for a while, and she played a magnificent role in Rob's healing journey.

Conclusion

When we are wounded, even before birth, we become little parents for our souls. We begin that process by caring at a deep level. We begin the process of caretaking. We develop coping mechanisms to protect ourselves. We begin to build hard shells to protect ourselves, to nest, and to cushion against the pain and hurt we find along the way. We begin to leave parts of the world as we know it, and we begin to construct our own worlds, all to protect ourselves.

When we begin to tell our stories, we begin to heal. It is not just the telling of these stories, it is also to whom they are told, who is listening, and how the stories are understood and supported— the contact with another human being, the presence and light of another set of human eyes. I believe the biggest contribution in therapy is the human contact with someone who understands the suffering, pain, struggles, hurt, and trauma of the human spirit or soul. I believe that when one set of human eyes meets another with love and compassion, that in itself is the healing. That is the true medicine, the spiritual energy. The Laika teachers call this spiritual medicine and say that it resides in us all.

A few months ago I visited Rob and Shelly and their two beautiful sons and two dogs in Toronto. We sat in their beautiful backyard, all of us just quietly reflecting. Then came that special moment in which we all uttered, "This is life. Indeed this is life."

Chapter Eleven

Life-Threatening Illness

Introduction

The diagnosis of a life-threatening illness can create extreme disruption in the life of most individuals and can throw anyone into turmoil. Such a diagnosis can be an immediate threat to one's general sense of peace and order and can represent a crisis. Most people walk around with the idea that cancer is associated with death, pain, and suffering.

When Debora received her breast cancer diagnosis, she fell into a state of shock and disbelief. I was out of the country when I received the first call from her doctor, Jenny Melamed. Dr. Melamed feared for Debora, as her large tumor appeared to be spreading. I did not respond to the call right away, but that night while I was asleep I heard a great voice saying to me softly, "Call Debora as soon as you can. She needs you." This woke me up and surprised me. Who was this powerful woman who could channel for help at such a long distance? I called the next day, and discovered that indeed she needed to hear a human voice that could support and help her right away.

As I listened to her I sensed her fear and emotional pain. I told her that I knew all would be well, and I shared my dream with her. I echoed to her that the Creator loved her so much and would be with her all the way. I encouraged her to cultivate a faith so strong that nothing negative could stand in the way of her surgery, her recovery, and all the other therapies to come. She said that she could do that and that she was strong in her faith, but she also asked the normal questions. "Why me? Why now? I just lost my husband to cancer three years ago. I have two young children. What will become of them?" I reassured and supported her as much as I could on the telephone, and we set up our first meeting.

The First Meeting

At the time of her diagnosis, Debora was a fifty-year-old Jewish widow with two young children. She had lost her husband three years before and was still in deep and painful mourning, as he had died just three and a half weeks after his diagnosis. This scared the hell out of Debora. Her doctor and personal friend referred her. She was waiting for the pathology results at the time, and she was tearful, scared, and anxious throughout that first session. She had an aged mother who was not well, and she was an only child. She feared that this news would destroy her mother, as she was also still grieving the loss of her only son-in-law.

Debora had already implemented many of the things that I suggested, such as looking into alternative therapies, remaining positive no matter what, focusing on the here and now, and cultivating a powerful prayer life and faith in herself, the Creator, and the strength of her mother and her children. We explored how she would inform her children, her mother, and her friends. One of the most important things that I stressed to Debora was to get as many friends and family as she possibly could to support and love her during this difficult time. (She did that right away. She contacted her best friend and confidante and many others, and they became her army of strength and hope.) At the end of the session, Debora was positive, determined, and ready to take things on as they presented themselves. I was astounded at her strength and her faith. Her fear of impending death dissipated.

By her second visit, she had received the test results, and they were not good. She would have to undergo six months of chemotherapy, a mastectomy, reconstructive surgery, and radiation therapy. She was devastated and said that she felt totally abandoned by God. She wept from a very deep place. She experienced a repeat of

121

all the traumatic events that she had endured during her husband's diagnosis and death. She was in a dark place and devoid of hope. We sat together quietly. I remember silently asking the Creator for words of hope, support, and healing to offer Debora.

Debora then remembered that she had had a dream about her late husband; it had been a very positive dream, and she had felt that he was with her. In that moment a change in the energy occurred. Indeed beautiful and powerful angels come forth in times of turmoil and pain, and in that session, we both felt that profound presence. I told Debora about the power of connecting with our ancestors as they walk with us through times of difficulty and pain, and I encouraged her to connect.

At the end of that session we had a plan set in motion that included the following elements:

1. Safety and self-care, the two most important ingredients for healing;
2. Thought tracking, that is, watching the ego mind and making sure that she took any negatives and turned them into positives;
3. Staying hopeful, as hope would be the driving force for her healing;
4. Engaging in exercise, maintaining a healthy diet, and losing weight;
5. Connecting with a naturopathic doctor;
6. Practicing deep breathing and breathing exercises;
7. Meditating, which we started right way;
8. Switching to eating only organic produce;
9. Journaling; and
10. Attending weekly healing sessions.

Debora again showed a strength and faith that could move mountains. As the weeks and months went by, I observed during every visit that Debora never uttered a negative word. She struggled, yes, like any other human being, but she was positive and had the most amazing humor. Even in the depth of all the uncertainty, she made me laugh the greatest belly laughs. We know from research data that there are positive outcomes when clients engage in laughter therapy and meditation. We sat together through many beautiful meditation sessions, which were both healing and revealing.

During one particular session, Debora looked really sad and stressed out. She told me that she had been looking at research and statistics regarding her prognosis and realized that she did not stand a good chance at all. I reminded her that she was not a statistic but a fighting human being and mother and that with her faith and her doing all the right things, she would do very well. I often told her that deep down I just knew this to be true. As with all gifted healers, there are things that I just know. I have no explanation for them, just a knowing.

Debora was back on track. She was looking good. She had lost a lot of weight, and she was looking younger by the day. She was aware of the deeper transformation that was taking place at all levels, physical, emotional, and spiritual. So many of her friends connected with her and supported her. Her mother took it well and was her great support. Her children became her strength and cheered her on. I could see that Debora had found meaning in her suffering. As Viktor Frankl states in his book *Man's Search for Meaning*, "We must never forget that we may also find meaning in life even when confronted with a hopeless situation, when facing a fate that cannot be changed." I knew that Debora had found the courage to change this personal tragedy into a triumph; she turned her pain and hurt into a positive fight for life and love. It was visible and palpable in every session.

Debora's Story in Her Own Words

Like so many others, I went on with my life with regular routines, growing up, going to school, getting a job, getting married, and developing a home with a family. Life was good and normal.

My first experience with extreme loss was the death of my father. It was hard but not unusual to lose a parent to illness and age. Life went on pretty much as before once we all adjusted to this loss. Then out of the blue, my husband died at a very early age, and I was left alone with two young people looking to me for comfort and understanding as to what their lives would now be like without their father. My life was turned on its head. I have no brothers or sisters, and my late husband was also an only child. We started off as a very small family, and our numbers were shrinking. What I am blessed with are friends that are always there to lend whatever support they can.

During that time, I remembered something that I had learned when in my early twenties. From one of those self-help books came one piece of advice that has helped me through many difficult times. I will share this with you: When you find yourself in a difficult situation, plan to solve it by thinking of the worst possible thing that could happen and devising a way to solve this. Your imagination is always worse than the reality, and therefore, once you are prepared for the worst, the worst never happens, and reality is easier. So this is what I did, I looked at what I needed to do to help my family through this both emotionally and financially. And together with my children, we did it! I'm not saying it was easy. We still had and continue to have tough times around this loss.

I was sitting in my doctor's office and hearing the doctor say, "You have breast cancer, and it is malignant." *No! There must be some mistake. Me? Cancer?* I was yelling inside myself. There it was—slapped in the face with my own impending mortality. *How do I tell my family? What will become of them?* So many different thoughts swirled in my head. It was surreal.

When I told my children, the first question they had was "Are you going to die?" At that moment, I said to myself, "I'm going nowhere yet. I need to be here to see my children married and hopefully help raise some grandchildren." That became my answer to them. But inside I was terrified that I would not be able to fulfill my promise to them.

One day, the phone call came that changed my inner struggles. It was Teresa. My fears seemed to subside as I spoke to her. I felt safe! Her strong spirituality was like a blanket that spread warmth over me in a very cold part of my life.

With Teresa and many friends in my arsenal, I began my fight against this insidious disease. I have learned for the first time in my life to take care of me. As I go through life now, there is always that albatross of doubt about the cancer coming back. But I learned that I am stronger than I ever thought, which is something I attribute to my mother, who at age ninety is a rock. As a survivor of the Holocaust, she had to be, as she calls it, a toughie. Her motto is to never give up and to keep on fighting to the last breath. I realize now, that I have been strongly influenced by this philosophy.

My father blessed me with his humor. Even to this day, more than fifteen years since he died, when people reminisce about him, the first thing they remember is his jokes and how he always made them laugh. When he was in the hospital for the last time, he was constantly joking with the staff. My mom and I told him to concentrate on his health instead of entertaining. His response was that this was the better way, as it was nicer to see smiling faces helping rather than sour faces.

I am definitely a product of both of my parents, and I hope that my children will carry on their legacy of strength and humor. I feel extremely fortunate to have my lovely but small family as well as truly good friends who have stood by me through all kinds of adversities. And finally I am so grateful that Teresa came into my life to help lead me out of my darkest hours back into the light of life.

Conclusion

The day Debora came with the good news that she was in remission at the end of the two years, that no cancer existed in her body, and that she was cured, we celebrated with prayer, laughter, and tears of joy! Do I believe in miracles? Yes, I do. Daily as a healer I witness miracles in people's lives. What an honor to be a witness to this love, hope, compassion, caring, faith, and joy. What an honor.

Debora brought me two gifts, blankets that she had made. She had taken up crocheting and was making these beautiful blankets for homeless women. One blanket was for me and was woven in all my favorite colors. The other she said was for all the people who would come and sit in that same chair where she had felt safe, loved, and cared for. She wanted every other human being to experience during therapy what she had.

I could tell you endless stories about the magic love blanket that Debora made for my office. Every single person who came for healing and wrapped himself or herself in the blanket Debora had made told me over and over how safe, cozy, loved, and warm they felt. All I did then was to share Debora's story with them. Through the telling of her story to other human beings I saw hope emerge where hope had been absent; I saw calm descend where there had been fear; I saw love where there had been hate.

Thank you, Debora, for all the gifts and love that you brought into my life and the lives of so many. In doing this work I believe that there is reciprocity. As long as we as healers and caregivers can remember this gift of reciprocity, we will never grow tired or weary. We will feel renewed by every human being we touch with love and kindness.

In the Xhosa language there is a word *ubuuntu*, which means, "You have what it takes to be human. You recognize that you exist only because others exist. You are gentle, compassionate, hospitable, caring for the welfare of others." Debora, you have ubuuntu!

Chapter Twelve

Is This Abuse?

Introduction

Repetition compulsion or enactment is a symptom that walks with trauma victims like a shadow. It is a behavior that plagued many clinicians, including Freud and Jung. In the area of addiction we see clearly how clients repeat the same behaviors over and over, getting the same results. A few years ago, when I was preparing for a workshop on trauma, I came up with an explanation I thought people in the general public would be able to understand. I presented this workshop in a First Nation reserve, and my words had a profound impact on the participants. They are included below:

Repetition Compulsion

I repeat the same thing over and over so that I can feel the pain.
In expressing and feeling the pain, I myself bear witness to the people that see my pain.
In my pain, I say to the people that see my pain, look this is how I hurt at the time when I was that child, I had no witness and no one who could come and help me. Now I have to show people around me the hurt so that they will really help me.
I bear witness to my own pain.
My symptoms and my pain is the telling of my own story.
This is my own correctional experience … I will repeat it until I am totally heard and then I will change.
When I am heard, validated and acknowledged, only then I let it go, because I then do not need it any more.

Initial Contact

Anne sent out a crisis call a few months after she fell into yet another abusive relationship. Anne had just come out of an abusive relationship and was drowning her sorrows, drinking in a pub. Then she met this man. He was very charming, caring, and supportive, and on that first night she poured her heart out to him. She told him her life story of abuse, rejection, and trauma. They became intimate on that night, and he became her rescuer. He was also a health care professional, which helped Anne to feel understood, supported, and validated.

During this time Anne was struggling with alcohol as a soother and talked about this to her newfound love. He was a habitual cannabis smoker and introduced Anne to this new "healing" drug. She liked it. It took the edge off and made her feel calm and good. Within a matter of months she was addicted to it and could not start a day without it. Then the trouble started. After our first few sessions I was inspired to write two poems, but I never had the opportunity to share them with Anne as she always presented with another crisis during our sessions. The right time never came. These two poems will inform you of the dramas and pain that unfolded in this short-lived relationship.

Is This Abuse?

Give me something to believe in please
These thoughts, words, experiences will not cease
They haunt me day and night; I am too tired to fight
Release me. Show me, please where is the light?

Is it true, did this happen, where is the love?
Yesterday I had it all, the joy, hope, and spirit from above
Yes, he told me I was pure, beautiful he held me
Now I feel dirty, used and abused—please let me be

I am now a victim of emotional abuse they say
I am so confused; I don't know night from day
My heart is hurting so, I feel so empty and alone
The pain persists; it hurts even when I am stoned

He introduced me to marijuana in a few days of our meeting
Weeks later I needed it to ease his verbal beatings
He took my weakness and he used it against me
He was charming, so caring and smooth I could not see
When I told him that I had a problem with booze
He told me drink up honey, you have got nothing to lose

Why did this happen to me? Oh it felt so right
Did I put the call out for abuse, please hear my plight
Why me? Why now? It's hard for me to understand
Did I deserve this? The relationship had been so grand

All my beliefs about the safety of this world have been shattered
I am now the crazy, jealous, addict girlfriend battered
How do I trust, discern, oh how will I ever know
This experience it is so painful, I cannot take another blow

I want to take revenge, hurt him I want to attack
Help me let out this anger; tell me what do I lack?
Now the tears, the pain the suffering so great
Will I ever recover from this depressed and fragile state?

Say something; please say one thing to give me hope
Of late, I cannot get out of bed; I don't know how to cope
Confusion, illusion, chaos, memories please leave me alone
Right now I will be happy just to turn into a stone

You have to understand; this man was so gentle and kind
He loved me, cared for me, supported me, and that is the bind
In the midst of his love, he was hiding amongst holy men
He taught me about friends, kindness, family community and Zen

I am so tired, it is hopeless, and this helplessness and sadness I feel
I want to die, disappear forever what is the big deal
If all of this is true, his lies, his anger and deceit
Then just tell me what to do, how do I avoid a repeat?

There Is Hope

Your story is so painful so familiar and very sad
You found your voice and you came for help for that I am glad
I listened to you with my heart; yes I can see that it hurt so deep
Let it out, release, cry, scream, tell your story it is good to weep

You are not alone anymore, you are here, and your words carry the
pain
You will heal from this; with healing you will remove the stain
I see your struggle, I sense the confusion and yes I know
Humans are capable of horrible deeds, I understand the blow

Just remember my dear that it was not your fault at all
Please praise yourself, be kind, you had the courage to make that call
At that time you thought that you were weak, you were so strong
What he did was very cruel, very painful, and also so wrong

You are beautiful, blissful, bountiful, courageous, intelligent and
more
It is hard, yet we have to name it, so that you can receive the balm for
the sore
Because of your naivety, your gentleness, kindness and all that love in
your heart
You easily fell prey to this manipulation and became a board for his
dart

You are brilliant, you figured it out and finally listened to your voice
Now you will learn, in this work that you always have a choice
You have to love yourself and keep safe, and take good care
In future always look deeply; it's all right to be aware
Sometimes for wolves that came dressed in sheep's attire
As you said very soon you discovered that he was a liar

Speak to your dear good friends, reach out if you can
It is hard, it feels new, and scary, can be awkward I understand
Try once and then take the risks, because we all need connection
On the healing journey you will experience correction

You are far more than your thoughts, your mind and the emotions
Your true identity, your essence, your higher self is greater than the ocean
You are not alone, connected to earth and ancestors you are
There is the soft smile, yes you are strong, and soon you will be a star

You are safe now; you have a witness and more
You will see in this pain, and struggle what is really in store
There are no mistakes in life only lessons to learn
Do the work, listen, look deeply and you will earn
You will trust again, love again, and respect self again
You will experience love, joy, truth the opposite of pain

Safety, self-care, self-love and care you will embrace
You can take your time; do the work at your own pace
Live in the here and now, mindfully and stay present always
Healing will come; you are protected by all the sunrays

Childhood Background

Anne never linked trauma and abuse to her situation. She thought that her behavior was something that most young women experienced, even after the history taking when I came up with the diagnosis of complex posttraumatic stress disorder. She kept asking the question (hence the title of her story), "Is this abuse?"

Anne was the oldest of four siblings; she had three younger brothers. Her mother was Pilipino and her dad Chinese. There were many cultural differences between her parents, and she was exposed to her father's discrimination and negative remarks against her mother for her entire life. It was clear that Anne's dad felt that he was better than her mother.

As a child she witnessed constant physical and verbal abuse between her parents, and she began to normalize this. The constant sexist discrimination by her father, including in his interactions with Anne and her brothers, became a norm for her. She was always treated differently, and she modeled the behavior of her mother. She became aware that mother always felt less than, and she felt the same.

One day during a session she shared her most painful childhood memory with me, which had its roots in an experience that happened many times during her growing up. Her parents were engaged in a physical and verbal fight. Her father was drunk at this time. Anne, about four and a half at the time, was watching from a distance, hiding as usual. When she saw blood, she went to her room and hid under her bed. She stayed there until the fight was over. When everything was quiet she came out and wet herself. She returned to bed in a fearful state. No one ever came to reassure her or explain anything to her. The next day things went back to normal—until the next time. By then Anne was already deeply traumatized.

As Anne grew older, she always confided in her parents about her relationships and turmoil but never received validation or support. Her father felt she had it coming to her. She left home at a very young age, studied, and completed a degree. She wanted to be a professional woman, unlike her mother who was oppressed by her father. She was highly intelligent, and when I met her, she was working as a journalist. She was beautiful, articulate, and honest. In spite of this, she was suffering from low self-esteem.

Healing Sessions

Anne was in the depths of dealing with a very traumatic relationship breakup. She had fallen head over heels for this man. They had spent most of their time with each other, practically living together. Initially it had been bliss. He had treated her well. He was into martial arts and meditation, and she was into yoga, which she loved, as it was one of her healing balms. They also smoked pot habitually and drank a lot of alcohol.

When Anne came to me, she was addicted to cannabis and was a problem drinker. During many of the sessions Anne would bring in a crisis situation, and we would deal with it. I spent many sessions educating Anne on addiction and trauma. I referred Anne to the Centre for Addiction and Mental Health, as she wanted to practice a harm-reduction approach. She was reluctant to give up the substances, as they were helping her to cope, but the other interventions (yoga, meditation, nutrition, breathing, grounding, focusing, and thought tracking) helped Anne as she struggled in the healing process. She was very angry and internalized this for a very long time, causing her to suffer with chronic depression. She was put onto antidepressants. During these sessions we also had to deal with separation and termination, as I was moving away to Vancouver. Anne still needed a lot of work but was making headway.

Work Relationships

Anne was very unhappy in her current position as a journalist and also had many stormy and conflict-filled work relationships. Trauma destroys sustaining bonds, and while the wounds are alive and active, trauma will infiltrate all aspects of life. While in therapy Anne became inspired to earn a master's degree in psychology. She researched and applied to programs and was accepted into one.

As the months went by, Anne became brighter and more positive, but she still had a long way to go. Healing from the amount to trauma she had endured would be a longer process. Anne was aware of this, and we began to talk about other therapists. Our journey ended when I left for Vancouver and Anne entered her master's program. We set up a few phone sessions for transition.

Comments

Many traumatized individuals constantly feel a profound sense of loneliness and alienation from others. To satisfy their need to belong, a need common to all people, traumatized individuals with shattered self-esteem, fears, and unmet needs for connection are at extremely high risk for gravitating toward the most readily available forms of social support: the crowd at the local tavern and drug-using party people. In Anne's case this reality was profound.

Anne presented with a number of psychological disturbances that resulted from severe childhood trauma. Posttraumatic symptoms often appear to be logical consequences of childhood abuse. Freud's repetition compulsion appears to be highly applicable to repressed childhood trauma, and adults with such backgrounds evidence many different ways of reliving experiences as well as avoidant symptoms and autonomic arousal. Anne suffered consequences of the failures of attachment and the inadequate care and protection that are common in dysfunctional and abusive families.

Many women seeking treatment for depression, suicidal feelings, substance use problems, difficult or abusive relationships, and self-inflicted harm may actually be experiencing complex posttraumatic stress response. Many health care professionals have little or no knowledge of or training in dealing with trauma and addictions. Clients report that in most settings neither disorder is attended to. Research now shows that the success of treatment depends on thorough assessment, information, and education at the initial contact for both disorders (Poole and Greaves 2007). This information and preparation immediately inform clients that clinicians acknowledge and understand the complexity of both disorders; thus both disorders are "owned" by clients, which encourages responsibility, collaboration, and a healthy therapeutic relationship from the outset.

Clinicians must be sensitive in the assessment phase. Diverse and gender-specific knowledge and insight are crucial. Some questions are extremely difficult for some women, and clinicians should inform clients about their choices up front. Honest, clear, and open communication is essential. Clinicians should also be aware of sudden disclosure of posttraumatic histories and the risk of relapse and further trauma.

Many self-destructive behaviors reenact trauma, particularly for the victims of childhood abuse, who represent a large segment of people with this dual diagnosis. These patients, even though the trauma and abuse occurred years ago, treat themselves in ways that repeat the severe abuse and neglect of their pasts; they treat themselves in the same ways that they were treated. In this way they repeat their own past experiences of pain and suffering thus ignoring their own needs.

Conclusion

The most crucial aspect of therapy is the development of a good therapeutic alliance. In Anne's case, our relationship was the key that opened the door to the work that needed to be undertaken. Healing lies within the therapeutic relationship. Issues of safety and trust are to be considered at all times. Women in particular bring with them their suffering, hurt, pain, guilt, shame, helplessness, and hopelessness, and through these symptoms they tell us how bad it was and still is. A compassionate, caring, and giving professional with deep knowledge and skills can support and assist women on their healing journeys.

Chapter Thirteen

Group Therapy for Trauma and Addiction

Introduction

Traumatic events destroy the sustaining bonds between individuals and their views of themselves, others, and the world. Trauma robs a person of his or her human connections and sense of community. Traumatized individuals often express or display that their sense of self-worth, of humanity, depends upon a feeling of connection to others. In my practice I hoped and believed that the solidarity of a trauma and addiction group could provide the strongest protection against terror and despair and hopefully the strongest antidote to traumatic experiences.

> *Trauma isolates.* The group creates a sense of belonging.
> *Trauma shames and stigmatizes.* The group bears witness and affirms.
> *Trauma degrades the victim.* The group exalts.
> *Trauma dehumanizes the victim.* The group restores humanity.

Dr. Judith Herman states that the above is factual and true and is experienced during powerful moments in group psychotherapy.

Background

I met Christopher Doyle during his psychiatric residency in Toronto. He wanted to do work with the most challenging psychiatric client population and also specialize in addiction psychiatry. He approached me one morning and said that he had had a conversation with his supervisor and wanted to work with me as a co-facilitator in one of my groups. He wanted to learn from me. In our discussion we shared our views, morals, beliefs, and values around working with people who suffered from both disorders. We soon learned that we shared similar views and philosophies. We believed that both disorders were deeply connected and that they should be treated simultaneously. We talked about the idea of establishing a group for clients with both disorders. We worked diligently on a proposal, and Christopher talked to his supervisor, Molyn Leszcz, head of psychiatry at Mount Sinai Hospital. Before we knew it, we were sitting together as co-facilitators in our first group for clients with trauma and addiction.

The group met once a week for ninety-minute sessions over a period of one year. It was a mixed-gender group of ten people—five males and five females—and it was also a closed group, meaning that all the members who started the group would end treatment at the same time. We did not admit new members. The facilitators had to meet with Molyn Leszcz once a week for supervision and teaching. I was ecstatic knowing that I was going to be supervised by one of the most respected psychiatrists in Canada.

In this chapter I will give you a snapshot of the group process during different stages of the group. My hope is that this information will be helpful and will shed light on the work involved with treating concurrent disorders. I also hope to encourage people who are fearful of groups to see the value in the treatment process.

A Model for Treatment

Here I will present a group treatment model for traumatized patients with addictions. My partners and I designed it to take into account the traumatic nature, the sequelae of abuse experiences, and struggles with addiction. We believed that group therapy had the potential to offer unique therapeutic benefit. Group participation reduces the intense isolation and sense of deviancy that traumatized and addicted individuals so frequently experience and find so distressing. Group therapy can validate the reality of the victimization and confirm affective experiences, which often are denied or distorted by the survivor and others in his or her family. At the same time, the disclosure of a powerful, burdensome secret in the presence of an empathic support group can provide enormous therapeutic relief.

In this group model we focus on difficulties these patients experience in relational skills, affect tolerance, behavioral control, self-identity, and self-worth.

1. In the early stage the focus is on building basic relational and coping skills, coupled with a great emphasis on self-care, safety, and goal clarification.

2. The middle stage of the group method focuses more on exploration and abreaction of traumatic experiences.

3. The late stage of the group method focuses on stabilization of gains and increased personal growth, particularly in relation to the external world. This does not occur as neatly and linearly as described but rather with rocking back and forth, movement between stages, relapse, and so on. The key to it all is that it is a safe place of acceptance.

Repeatedly in the testimony of traumatized individuals, there comes a moment when the sense of connection is restored by another person's unaffected display of generosity. Something that the victim believes to be irretrievably destroyed within himself or herself—faith, decency, courage, or a similar quality—is reawakened by a demonstration of common altruism. Mirrored in the action of others, the survivor recognizes and claims a lost part of himself or herself. At that moment, the survivor begins to rejoin the human community. (Yalom 1985). This was beautifully demonstrated in one of the group sessions I co-facilitated.

Case Example: Session Four

During check-in time, Len sat with his leg in a cast elevated on another chair. Christopher asked Len about his leg. (In this act, Christopher noticed, observed, acknowledged, and took care of Len.) He told us that he had fallen. Then he said, "I want to kill myself. I am so despondent. How long will all this carry on?"

"Why would you want to kill yourself?" Chris asked. He said that he did not feel good about himself and that he did not deserve to get anything good. This comment was met with silence. We listened and attended. He then continued his story. He said that he had met a woman, a beautiful human being. His face became soft and gentle as he spoke of her. She did not use drugs or alcohol, and he described her as loving and caring. She had been so wonderful to him, cleaning his apartment, cooking for him, and caring for him. He told us that he did not know how to deal with this love and care; he felt that he did not deserve it.

Carl said, "In my opinion it is a good thing that is happening to you, but it is all so rushed and all so soon. Just be careful—I am happy for you, but I do not want you to get hurt." This was mistrust, coupled with support and validation, very genuine and good.

Adam said, "Wow! You should be feeling good—send her to me." There was some envy and loneliness on his face. James commented, "It is marriage for sure." He laughed. In his own way James almost disengaged from the group. Len said that he knew all that was being said to him, but that his entire state of mind was fear, mixed with some good feelings.

Teresa asked, "What is it that you fear? Can you tell us more?"

"It's good," Len answered. "It feels good when someone does something for you, but the fear is about rejection." Some members commented and validated this fear. They further encouraged Len to take the risk. He said that he felt so much better after sharing and expressing his feelings.

Comments

To witness this process as it happens is indeed powerful. Len had the opportunity to explore his fears and to share his joy. He received undivided attention, honesty, and trust from the group and the leaders. He experienced the support. With exploration he realized that it was okay to share his fear. He was in touch with his most honest, sincere, gut-level feelings, thus he could also experience joy in the presence of genuine, caring, and loving people. I believe that we took him to a place where the parents (so to speak) played the vital role of telling the child that it was okay and safe to go out and love other people, that it was risky but also safe. This was the power of that moment, a glimpse of human transformation in a group.

The restoration of social bonds begins with the discovery that we are not alone. Nowhere is this experience more immediate, powerful, or convincing than in a group. Irvin Yalom, an authority on group psychotherapy, calls this the experience of universality. (Yalom 1985). The therapeutic impact of universality is especially profound for people who have felt isolated by shameful secrets. Because traumatized people feel so alienated by their experiences, groups have a very special place for them in the recovery process. The encounter with others who have undergone similar trials dissolves feelings of isolation, shame, and stigma.

Reenactment

Groups have proved invaluable for trauma of extreme situations. Participants repeatedly describe their solace in simply being present with others who have endured similar ordeals. Often re-experiencing trauma and pain through story telling can evoke painful emotions in the entire group. This can often prove to be the most challenging aspect of this model for the therapist. The key here is to modulate or regulate and thus bring the emotions down. The principle involved here is containment and metabolizing, as depicted in the next example.

Case Example: Session Seven

One day, about halfway through a session, when some of the members had gone for a smoke, Carl told a brutal story. He had received a fifteen-year prison sentence for robbing a bank. At that time he was a full-blown drug addict and alcoholic. He had robbed this bank with other drunken friends, and they had gotten away with two hundred thousand dollars. They crossed the border and ended up in the United States. Carl told some drug dealers at a bar that the group had two hundred thousand dollars in their room, and the dealers robbed them of the money. Carl turned himself in and returned to Canada. When he received his sentence, he told the judge that he was acting out with his friends and had been under the influence of alcohol. He also told the judge that he would never stop drinking, and the judge sentenced him to fifteen years imprisonment. Carl was in deep pain as he told his story. He stated that he did not want to end up in prison. In that moment, he also realized how much of his behavior was acting out. He saw that he had been looking for attention, and he realized that he always looked for attention in negative ways.

In prison much bigger men physically, verbally, and sexually abused him. On one occasion an inmate pushed his head through the prison bars and brutally raped him. He sustained a fractured skull and lost most of his teeth, and his eye was hanging out. Carl was now in deep pain as he told us why he feared men. He said that he had initially been fearful of Christopher but was slowly overcoming it. Despite the emotional pain, Carl appeared relieved to talk about it. Christopher asked him how he was feeling. "Still fearful and in pain but relieved." Carl answered. "I never shared this story before today."

He also added that he was really trying to take good care of himself. Just then, James and Adam returned from the smoke break. Christopher, Len, and I were still shaken by Carl's recounting of this brutal experience. Len was quiet and thoughtful. I told James and Adam about the disclosure and that it was important for them to hear the story. Christopher briefly retold the story. It was a powerful moment because, as Christopher was telling the story, he also repeatedly told the group how difficult it must have been for Carl. He thus again validated Carl's pain and current feelings. It felt so good and so right.

I told Carl that I fully understood now why he had been so frightened when James had had an aggressive outburst in a previous group session. James said that his anger was still contained and that it was nothing. Carl said that he understood where the anger was coming from, but that it had been truly scary for him all the same. James became very quiet and sat back in his chair. Both Christopher and I again supported Carl. Adam and Len remained very quiet.

Then James interjected in a loud voice, "You did not give me the opportunity to give Carl feedback about my feelings." He then proceeded to tell Carl about his feelings and what it had been like for him on the day that he had had the aggressive outburst. He also told Carl that he was very sorry. I told James that I was sorry for interjecting, that I really valued his honesty, and that he had tremendous strength and courage.

We called the session to a close. I validated the pain, affect, honesty, and courage experienced in the group that day and asked members to give their feedback. Carl was relieved that he had shared his story and said that he realized that there were still so many feelings hidden. Len commented that he found the group helpful and was feeling so much better. James was okay and ready to leave the room. Adam said he was feeling fine. Christopher talked to the group about alternative ways to deal with their anger and feelings and explored briefly the topic of self-care. He also validated their current self-care and their bringing their honest and painful emotions to the group.

The Debrief

Christopher and I felt that it had been an excellent session. "Finally, we are working," he said. We processed well and contained and metabolized the feelings and emotions. We briefly talked about our reaction to Carl's horrible story. I was exhausted and experienced pain in my chest. Christopher was very supportive and said that if I needed to talk later, I should call him.

Supervision with Dr. Molyn Leszcz

Molyn stated that the group content was highly emotional and that we had done well with regulating the emotions and pain in the group. Many painful experiences and issues were explored during that session; and Molyn supported us and commented that we must have been exhausted after such an intense session. It was good to get that feedback. Both Christopher and I would never have survived the group without the supervision and support from Molyn.

Comments

With deep sharing, pain, and suffering comes growth. The development of intimacy and cohesion emerges, and a complex mirroring process comes into play. The presence of skilled and competent leaders who have a very good relationship and an understanding of each other's worldview and view of self can only enhance this process. It is mandatory to be able to contain, modulate, and regulate affect with one's presence and support in the here and now.

As group members extend themselves to each other, they become more capable of receiving the gifts that others have to offer. The tolerance, warmth, love, and compassion they grant to others begins to rebound. Though this type of mutually enhancing interaction can take place in any relationship, it occurs most powerfully in the context of a group. Yalom describes this process as an adaptive spiral in which group acceptance increases each member's self-esteem and each member in turn becomes more accepting toward others. (Yalom 1985). Again this does not happen in isolation or without direction but with the wit and skill of the group's leaders.

Risks in Groups and Limit Setting

The destructive potential of groups is equal to their therapeutic promise. We must not be naive about this point. The role of group leader carries with it the risk of the irresponsible exercise of authority. Conflicts can erupt within the group, with members assuming the roles of perpetrator, accomplice, bystander, victim, and rescuer. Such conflicts can be hurtful to individuals and can lead to group demise.

Case Example: Session Twenty-Three

During this particular session, everyone was struggling. Ken was checking in when James became extremely agitated. James asked Ken to hurry so that we could carry on with the group. Tension was present and palpable in the room.

Millie had had a difficult week. She described periods of dissociation and used the term "losing time" (almost as though she had left her body with no memory of it or the events that transpired during those moments). She expressed her fear about this and described a few very frightening experiences, including waking up in her mother's house without knowing how she had gotten there.

Christopher asked Millie if she knew what was happening to her. He offered a brief psychoeducational blurb on dissociation. He explored the issue with her and asked her why she thought the dissociation had begun happening recently. Christopher then referred back to James's question to Millie two weeks ago about her father. Loaded with emotion, she told the group on this day that her father had been the perpetrator of her trauma, but she stopped the abuse. This took a great amount of energy, and the tension continued to mount.

Members of the group gave Millie feedback. Leo, James, and Sam shared their experiences with dissociation. Millie thus received very little support from the group. It was as if the group could not be empathic, and they appeared to be devastated and crippled by Millie's disclosure.

Ken gave Millie an empathic response, stating how sorry he was. Then he said, "I am sick and tired of members playing games."

"Millie was disclosing serious abuse issues, and we could not be there for her. We did not even lay the ground or prepare for this," Leo said.

I asked, "Leo, how would you have liked this group to go?"

"I want people to be sensitive, to talk about their honest feelings and needs, and to work on their abuse issues."

"How could we have dealt better with all the issues that came up today, and how are we going to close this group?" I asked.

Helen expressed her concern for Millie and told the group that they had not stayed with Millie and had failed her.

"How can we help Millie right now?" I asked. Christopher very gingerly began talking about the importance of open, honest, and clear communication.

We then told the group that it was time for closure, so each member spoke. Helen very empathically supported Millie and said that it had been a difficult group.

"The group was a tremendous challenge today for everyone," I said. "So much happened and so many good things, too. Honesty was present, and old unresolved issues were brought up again; and that was good, too," I explained. I validated the group by saying, "It takes courage to put our fingers in our wounds. The group worked hard and struggled, but I now sense calm and support."

Ken was feeling better. Millie said that she was very anxious and fearful. She was now reassured and supported. Adam said listening to Millie today brought up some issues about his own abuse. "This is what group is all about, open and honest communication. I am feeling so much better now," said Leo.

Supervision with Dr. Molyn Leszcz

Molyn stated that in order to be successful, a group must have a clear, focused understanding of its therapeutic task and the structure that protects all participants adequately against the dangers of traumatic reenactment and victimization. He said that this work is rooted in the fundamental and core principles. He emphasized that our interventions emerge from responsibility, self-care, affect/emotion regulation, and sobriety.

Dealing with Relapse in a Group

Case Example: Session Thirty

Millie had a few drinks before group. She was intoxicated, laughing as she asked the group whether she could stay. Ken was very angry and confronted her. The rest of the group gave her feedback and told her she could stay for the session. She opened up and talked about how she was in turmoil and in pain. She then started to beat herself up. She said that she really wanted to stop using, that she would like to sober up. She also commented that she felt supported by the group.

Various group members gave very authentic and honest responses. James supported Millie and also showed his own vulnerability in the process. He was hurting, and he articulated this and showed the group. His pain was present and palpable. Sheila shared some of her abuse issues yet remained very supportive toward Millie. Sam talked about his abuse as well but was also very supportive toward Millie. Carl encouraged Millie. Throughout this session the entire group showed profound love and care, yet the members also exposed their own struggles and vulnerability.

Supervision with Dr. Molyn Leszcz

"When a member arrives at group intoxicated, it's a tricky situation," Molyn explained. "We have to remain open and honest, and we have to continue to set limits and boundaries. It has to be put out there, in the open, in the most honest and supportive way," Molyn further stated. "The exploration of the group norms needs to be revisited at this time."

We had talked about the situation openly and questioned the meaning of this behavior for the group. We explored what was acceptable to the group as well as exploring the behavior of that member. Why had she brought herself to the group intoxicated? We also explored acceptance by the group and acting out. We finally helped them make a bad situation better. The group offered love and support. We held; we contained the group. Molyn further stated that when a member comes to the group intoxicated, we have an opportunity to explore the situation and the person the way they really are in their struggle.

Conclusion

At the end of the year, seven members out of the ten completed all sessions. This was an amazing retention. The group was a great success in the way that we defined *success*. For the purpose of this group and work, I term it successful because almost all members became clean and sober and began to join society and life in the world. Deep connections developed among members, and both Christopher and I continued to support them in their individual work. During the cycle of the group, we also offered all the group members individual sessions. One of the most important aspects of this work was case management. Molyn stated that without case management the group would never have survived.

Just as the body can be traumatized, so can the psyche or the spirit. On the psychological and mental levels, trauma refers to the wounding of one's emotions, spirit, will to live, dignity, sense of security, and beliefs about oneself and the world.

The wounded child contains:

- Damaged patterns of childhood and youth;
- Painful memories;
- Negative attitudes from the past;
- Negative modeling;
- Dysfunctional images; and
- Negative relational patterns.

We take all of these dysfunctional patterns into our adult life and live through these wounds. (For example, the fear of abandonment is played out through jealousy.) In psychotherapy we call this repetition compulsion. We repeat these patterns through sex, addiction, alcoholism, smoking, obsessive fear of failure, helplessness, and hopelessness; and we become the people who mistreated us. When we internalize our oppression, we live through our wounds.

These responses lead to

- Damage to self and the relationship with self;
- Damage to others and our relationships with others;
- Damage to our family, personal, and professional lives;
- Damage to our health;
- Damage to society; and
- Damage to the world.

During the life of the group, all of the above were addressed in the most profound, supportive, and authentic manner. With our presence and caring, we allowed all of the members to experience emotional correction. Through the new knowledge, insight, and support, they healed their deep-seated wounds. They could enter the world and relationships without their wounds.

I learned, grew, and transformed into a better person, caregiver, and clinician through my work with this group. Christopher became a more giving, loving, and caring doctor because of this work. My heartfelt thanks and love go out to my teachers, that is, all of the people in this group as well as Christopher and Molyn.

Chapter Fourteen

Death of a Group Member

Introduction

The anxiety, fear, and uncertainty of a diagnosis of cancer or some other life-threatening illness can leave individuals and families devastated, lost, and in turmoil. The many who have walked this journey say that after being diagnosed with cancer, one's life is never the same again. Death creates chaos. Moreover, it creates a sense of bafflement through a moral paradox: Questions that emerge would be why me? Why at this time in my life? In addition to the loss of life itself, client's major fears are of being in pain, forgotten, abandoned, alone, and shamed in the sense of not living or dying in the proper manner or with integrity. I promised John on his deathbed that I would write and share his story with the world. He wanted me to do this.

All people—the dying and the bereaved—experience grief as a response to death. *Grief* is the affective or emotional response caused by a significant loss of something or someone important to a person. From one person to the next, grief differs in intensity and the duration of time needed to resolve the loss. *Bereavement* is the term used to refer to the experiences that follow the death of a loved one, and *mourning* is the term used to describe the social customs and cultural practices that follow a death.

The fears that accompany the client and family are real, normal reactions to a new diagnosis, a crisis, or devastating news. Death of a loved one or facing one's own death can immobilize our strengths and increase our fears.

149

What follows in this chapter is a description and discussion of the impact of the diagnosis and/or death of a member in a group established to provide support and psychotherapy for individuals with concurrent mental health and substance use disorders. I will explore the group process and dynamics and interventions by the group therapist. The chapter further explores a case-illustrated journey by a nurse, John, a very compassionate human being who helped and touched the hearts of many clients and professionals as he embarked upon dealing with his diagnosis and addiction, his suffering and grief, and as he challenged the medical and nursing profession to take a look at our management of this most vulnerable population.

Cigarette smoking is one of the most preventable health hazards of modern times. According to the American Cancer Society, cigarette smoking is related to four hundred thousand deaths in the United States each year. Despite intensive documentation of its risks, many people continue to smoke cigarettes or use smokeless tobacco (Centers for Disease Control 1994). Tobacco is the primary cause of many cancers (including lung, oral, pancreatic, cervical, kidney, and bladder), and accounts for more than 29 percent of all cancer deaths in the United States (American Cancer Society 1997).

Group Psychotherapy for Clients with Cancer

The use of group psychotherapy as a modality for the psychological support and treatment of clients with cancer is well documented. The literature describes various types of groups, in terms of both the composition of such groups and the use of different types of psychotherapeutic strategies. A survey of the literature indicates that, as might be expected, in those groups containing clients with advanced disease, the topic of death and dying emerges frequently and predictably (Corey 1996). By contrast, little has been written on how to deal with or discuss the issue of death and dying in homogenous time-limited groups, especially when the client's cancer is in an early curable stage.

Group Psychotherapy for Addiction

The therapy approach offered to patients in the groups included a modified dynamic group therapy (MDGT) and principles of interactional group psychotherapy. The interactional group therapy process is built on the concept that the group is more than the sum of its parts. That is, the interpersonal interaction of group therapy participants assumes a therapeutic dynamic that can only occur when there are several participants. For this reason, group therapy generally involves eight to ten patients. Newly arriving patients join existing groups, allowing patients in early treatment to observe a progressive mental clearing in other clients in later stages of treatment. This group therapy differs from self-help and other support groups by the presence of a therapist or facilitator. Group therapy of this type may involve one or two facilitators.

The conceptual basis of MDGT differs from early psychodynamic psychotherapy in its basic theoretical assumption and in the understanding and treatment of substance abusers. Psychodynamic psychotherapy originally stressed instinctual striving, conflict, and pleasure seeking. The MDGT approach emphasizes the developmental and structural impairments that have affected the capacities for self-regulation in an individual with substance dependence. What is quite evident and problematic is the addict's self-medication of psychological suffering. In contrast to psychodynamic theorists, the MDGT model also recognizes and emphasizes the strengths and restorative capacities of the addict that make therapy and recovery possible. The MDGT model regards the client as wounded but also as one who has a psychological foundation that is sufficiently intact to build upon. In MDGT the focus is on creating an atmosphere of safety and support where individuals learn about themselves and the way their character structure works. The importance of structure, continuity, and empathy is stressed to further encourage and engage clients. An active, friendly therapist leads these cohesive groups.

Members are encouraged to discover and to explore alternative ways of seeing, experiencing, and making choices.

Group leaders further ensure safety and comfort, and focus on feelings, relationships, self-esteem, and self-care. Clarification and interpretation are provided; and empathy, involvement, and support are encouraged. Focus is on support by the therapist. Themes that arise include peer pressure for abstinence from alcohol and drugs; the concept of universality; better understanding of struggles with addictions; understanding of attitudes and the confrontation of disabling ones; and creation of an awareness of pathological defense styles that prevent healthy and intimate relationships. Encouragement is offered to maintain healthy interpersonal relationships. Clients value the group for:

- Giving them feedback on their interpersonal behavior;
- Allowing them opportunities to express their repressed emotions;
- Allowing them to feel less isolated;
- Providing a sense of acceptance from other people;
- Improving their self-esteem by allowing them to help others;
- Helping them to discover unconscious motivations for their behavior; and
- Giving them feelings of optimism through the experience of watching others improve and leave treatment.

The client who died, John, was a core member of such a group. When he joined the group the group had already met for seven weeks.

Description of the Client who Died

When he joined the group, John had been diagnosed with early stage cancer of the larynx and had completed a six-week course of radiation therapy. He was a sixty-six-year-old, Caucasian, homosexual male. He lived with his partner for many years until his death two years prior to John's cancer diagnosis. John had a longstanding history of alcohol and tobacco addiction and received treatment for his alcohol addiction for many years at CAMH. John had long periods of abstinence from alcohol lasting up to fifteen years and from tobacco lasting up to ten years. John made a total career change at the age of forty. He had been an administrative clerk for many years and decided, after a long hospitalization for severe pancreatitis, to give back to the medical and nursing profession. He entered college and completed his RN certification after three years. After his graduation he started work as a staff nurse in a surgical unit. The last twenty years of his life had been dedicated to nursing. John was so proud of his endeavors and always talked about his career with a very special fondness. He loved his work.

Two years prior to John's death, Dr. David Marsh referred John to my care. Dr. Marsh was taking care of John's physical symptoms of withdrawal from alcohol. John had relapsed with his alcohol use after the death of his partner. Dr. Marsh believed that John was depressed, grieving, very lonely, and isolated. John began group psychotherapy coupled with bi-monthly individual sessions.

Throughout his participation in the group, John shared his honest feelings, fears, and struggles regarding his adjustment after the death of his partner. He started to deal with his isolation and loneliness and received tremendous support from the group. As his depression lifted, he became one of the most giving, empathic, and caring members. The group also encouraged him to focus on his own needs.

He helped many of the members who were struggling with their addiction, and he modeled his own sobriety and other longstanding periods of abstinence. He was a great cook and baked the most delicious cookies and cakes, not only spoiling the group but also always bringing enough for all the other staff members. He was also a very active member of his church; he could cross-stitch and make beautiful ornaments and would donate all his work to the church to raise funds. Very soon after this group ended, John was diagnosed with recurrent cancer, and he continued to see me on a monthly basis for support.

John told me the sad news of his diagnosis late one Friday afternoon, exactly a week after the group ended. He was still in shock and devastated by the news. He had just taken an early retirement package and had many plans for the future. He wept as he shared his fears, anxieties, and uncertainties and asked many questions. I supported him and remained honest and up front. He really appreciated this and often told me so. He also relapsed with his alcohol use and was still smoking about forty-five cigarettes a day. He said that he would stop when he was ready. At this time I suggested that John join another group that had started six weeks earlier.

Before entering the group, he went to the medical clinic at CAMH for detoxification and stopped using alcohol but continued to smoke. Then he asked me to walk him to the smoking clinic. With the care and support of a very caring physician, he stopped smoking after three weeks. He said that he wanted to leave this world, this life, clean and sober.

The Group Process

From the outset, John had been a highly valued member of the group. He had years of experience with his addiction and also many years of abstinence. He thus had a greater capacity and ability to explore these avenues with honesty and openness. The group was just moving into the middle phase, but generally, members shared personal information about their addictions and other mental health issues. Goals that emerged during this stage were around drug, harm-reduction, and financial issues. Various coping strategies were employed.

This was the first time that the group was confronted by a member's disclosure of a life-threatening illness. John's disclosure was initially met with shock, disbelief, and fear. Many questions were asked about the disease, cure, remission, and therapy. The group remained supportive toward John. They shared their own fears and current behaviors with drugs and tobacco. The group members applauded John for his openness, courage, and strength. The news had a tremendous impact on members of the group; some of those who had previously showed a lack of empathy or exhibited selfish behavior became very caring and supportive.

The co-facilitators were two master's level students in psychology, and this process became an excellent learning opportunity for them. They displayed their knowledge, skill, and support at all levels.

I was challenged at all levels as a group leader. The complexity of issues that emerged was enormous. John started to complain of pain and feared that the disease had returned. A few weeks later he was diagnosed with another squamous cell tumor of the larynx. This time the disease was more extensive. John again struggled with the news and shared his fears in the individual sessions to follow. He was confronted with the option of major extensive surgery and a permanent stoma. He could not receive radiation therapy again since he had received his total permitted dosage the first time around.

John courageously explored all the options during individual therapy. He missed a few group sessions during this time. He explored his current life status and looked at his future quality of life. We explored end-of-life issues in detail. This was indeed a very trying and stressful time for John. After a few discussions with the radiation therapist and oncologist, he opted for palliation. He could not imagine himself in a hospital bed after major surgery, dependent on others, and he wanted to die with dignity and respect. The doctors said that he had just a few months to live. John asked me to inform the group about this sad news and tell the members that he would join the group the following week. He handed this task over with assurance and strength. At this time John was abstinent from alcohol and tobacco; he again told me that he wanted to leave this life with a clear mind and in a dignified manner.

The Group's Reaction

The group was now in the middle phase, and most of the members were abstinent and working hard on different issues. I informed the group of John's decision and his prognosis and received many different reactions. Initially my announcement was met with a long silence and many sad and questioning facial expressions. This was followed with questions and comments pouring out from the group members' hearts and souls. The group expressed their own fears, anger, compassion, caring, and love.

I indicated that John had asked me to deliver the news with the message that he needed our support over the next few months; he trusted us and was allowing us into his suffering world and inviting us to be part of his journey. I added that John was in control and had made these choices himself, which took a lot of strength and courage. He chose how to live and also how to die.

I introduced the group once more to the subject of death and dying. Members shed tears and voiced their concerns and fears as they began to explore their own mortality and their current lives. The group moved to a deeper level. The honesty and vulnerability exposed was phenomenal. As the group leader I made sure that everyone was doing okay. I went around the room and asked each person individually how he or she was doing. I was moved with awe as the group members began a deeper dialogue into their own souls. They explored, questioned, and gave one another support and feedback. The entire group echoed that they would give John all the support he needed in the weeks and months to come.

During the next few sessions, John joined the group and addressed his impending death with dignity. He further explored his sadness, pain, and disappointments. He began to grieve his secondary losses. The group members verbalized their feelings and their compassion. They applauded his courage and honesty.

Some members even asked questions about punishment and moved the group into discussion of spirituality and God. John told the group that he had been given a life and had chosen to smoke and use alcohol. He did not believe in punishment but rather in the consequences of human behavior. He shared his spirituality and his relationship with God. He told the group that his God loved and that his faith had been his source of strength throughout his life and that this same faith was now sustaining him. He was also fully supported by his church.

Termination

Termination is often a very painful experience for group members. This group's termination was coupled with the impending death of a group member. As John brought the stages of mourning to the group, I modeled and facilitated the process.

Task One: Accepting the Reality of the Loss

All of the group members confronted their own pain, fears, anxieties, and sadness and explored them as a whole. They further searched their souls as John courageously explored his journey with the group. The loss was accepted at an intellectual and emotional level.

Task Two: Working Through the Pain of Grief

This task was again met with courage as John and the other members explored their pain and hurt at various levels. Witnessing this process in the here and now was indeed powerful. I led the group by encouraging honesty, modeling my own fears, and expressing my sadness and pain. John told the members about his funeral plan and the type of service he wanted. Some members asked if they could attend. This process was met with the deepest honesty, compassion, respect, and love.

Task Three: Adjusting to an Environment in which the Deceased Is Missing

The ending of this group was a bittersweet event. John baked cookies, and we had all sorts of other treats. He presented each member with a bookmarker that he had personally cross-stitched. The markers carried our initials. He also wrote personal letters to some of the members, particularly those who were still struggling with their addictions. The letters encouraged members to continue to try—to live and not to give up. This event was again met with the deepest honesty, courage, and empathy. As I observed this event I gave thanks and was humbly moved to be a participant and a witness. I experienced the difference in the termination of this particular group. John's impending death had given this group renewed strength, faith, and hope. They were thankful for so many things. They were now all abstinent; and they all expressed a deep appreciation for life. The issues of separation at the end of the group also focused members on applying new coping strategies to issues of loss.

After the group ended, most members continued to see me on a monthly basis. John and I met on a weekly basis. John's condition deteriorated quite rapidly. He became more fatigued and sometimes struggled with pain management. Every session was initiated with openness and honesty. The sessions were indeed challenging, and John had the opportunity to face and explore his fears, pain, and suffering in a supportive, honest, and accepting environment. He had my trust, respect, and support. He was in touch with his most honest, sincere, and gut-level feelings.

During this process John discovered that he was not alone. He received support from the medical staff at CAMH, his church, and his friends. He explored his finances and possessions with me and started to give things away to close friends and the church. He finally decided to leave most of his money to the church. He celebrated this decision. He stated at one point that he was feeling weak physically but strong emotionally, as he was empowered and in control of his life. John died peacefully in a palliative care unit two and a half months after the group ended.

John asked his best friend to call me and left her with a message to pass on to me. In the message he stated that he had tremendous respect for my integrity and honesty, and he sent all his blessings. He also asked me to come to the funeral and complete my work. I was to inform all the group members about his death. Due to the short notice, only one member could make it to the funeral; however, group members expressed their condolences, and they all had a sense of peace and completion. I had the same feeling. We all finished our unfinished business. They had walked a beautiful journey with this most courageous man. I shed a few tears but walked through the funeral with a sense of peace and tremendous strength. I also sensed John's spiritual presence, and I whispered to him that I would tell his story.

This man's life, personality, and generosity were celebrated at his funeral. There existed a deep sense of community. His colleagues loved and respected him. I felt honored and humbled to have been a part of this man's life.

John inspired me to embark upon my private practice in trauma and addiction, psychosocial oncology, and palliative care. He further challenged me to embrace oncology nursing once again and to say yes to my calling. He urged me to continue to teach these skills to other health care professionals.

Every loss is a death, and when we are confronted with death, we have to move through the process of grieving and mourning, and then we heal and grow.

Conclusion

With deep pain, sharing, and suffering comes growth. Our experiences with John had a deep impact on our lives as clinicians. Dr. David Marsh is my partner in life and shared this journey both professionally and personally. John had the deepest love and respect for David. During John's last days, David and I visited him in his home and in the palliative care unit. I watched their interaction, man to man, with awe. John would talk with David like a brother, and David remained so humble and transparent. He never hid his tears and fondness from John.

This process could only have been enhanced by the presence of skilled and competent leaders who had a sound knowledge base, solid skill set, and deep understanding of the nature of the human spirit and soul and of life and death. In this life we are constantly exposed to small deaths. With each loss or death comes the knowledge, wisdom, and understanding of ourselves and the people around us.

In reviewing the process notes, I was struck by how such major events in the life of the group could occur as one member brought his impending death to the rest. The fact that death had been so openly discussed had a tremendous impact on this group. Yalom and Grooves (1977) and Spiegel, Bloom, and Yalom (1981) have described support groups for clients with advanced cancer. They found that a sharing of anxieties concerning death and dying greatly detoxified the topic; they also found that involvement in the fellow member's death and dying greatly lessened the other members' fears and improved the overall morale of the group. The literature on groups for homogenous clients with early stage disease, however, has a great deal less to say about death and how it should be approached. There is evidence that each stage of the disease brings with it different concerns, and that death as a concern, while always present, does not usually get articulated as such until later in the client's illness.

In terms of this group, death and dying were not expected to be addressed as part of the group's agenda. When confronted with it, we had limited time, and the client and the leader gave members permission to deal with the issues in a very healthy and caring way. The group appreciated this, and they also continued to address all the other issues. Honesty, trust, compassion, understanding, and safety are core ingredients required for such work and dialogue, and they were all present most of the time.

As each member extended herself or himself to the others, each person became more capable of receiving the gifts and knowledge that others had to offer. The tolerance, warmth, love, and compassion they granted to each other was reciprocated. This was evident throughout the life cycle of this group; the mutually enhancing interaction was present and palpable. Yalom describes this process as an adaptive spiral in which group acceptance increases each member's self-esteem, and each member in turn becomes more accepting toward others.

Comments

Alcohol, tobacco, and other drugs (ATOD) play a major role in carcinogenesis through their effects on the entire body, including the immune system. Despite intensive documentation of the risks of these substances, many people continue to use. Health care professionals in clinics, addiction centers, hospitals, and the community at large face a multitude of problems and challenges presented by these clients daily. Add any medical problem or life-threatening illness such as cancer to the above and the clinician is confronted with the complexity of sorting out treatment and management. The effects of addiction are evident in the physical, psychological, social, emotional, and spiritual realms of these clients. This growing addiction and cancer pandemic has tested and challenged all human services.

Client and health care staff education is necessary because of the complexity of issues surrounding the care that is needed when clients present with concurrent medical and health issues. The sciences of pain management, cancer treatment, and treatment of addiction are all in the process of evolving.

A need exists for continued research in this field, as the number of addicted patients with cancer and terminal illness increases. Keeping clients informed and letting them participate in decision making will reduce anxiety and improve quality of life and psychological well-being.

Afterword: Notes from the Author

How does the soul respond when a task she has given is completed? At the end of writing this book, I had many mixed emotions: elation, relief, peace, sadness, exhaustion, love, joy, and pride.

I had made a commitment to my ancestors, the Creator, and myself to give the world a gift of deep healing and inner peace, the core reason for writing this book. Those hopes and dreams are woven into every word, experience, poem, and story. The book in itself now has a soul, or many souls connected as one with love and healing. Within the heart of this book resides a truth, surrounded by serenity, peace, and love. I extend those gifts to my fellow human beings with the hope that the book will deliver the elixir, balm, and medicine as promised.

The only real solution to all the hurt, trauma, and pain in the world is the healing power of love, forgiveness, truth, and the acceptance of others—partners, family, friends, community, and the world.

Namaste

Teresa Naseba Marsh

References

Chapter One: Trauma and Addiction

Bass, E. and Davis, L. *The Courage to Heal: A Guide for Women Survivors of Child Sexual Abuse.* New York: Harper & Row Publishers, 1988.

Bollard, K. 1990. A model for the treatment of trauma-related syndromes among chemically dependent women. *Journal of Substance Abuse Treatment.* 7, 83–87.

Brady, K. T., Killeen, T., Saladin, M. E., Dansky, B., and Becker, S. 1994. Comorbid substance abuse and posttraumatic stress disorder: Characteristics of women in treatment. *American Journal on Addictions.* 3:160–164.

Breslau, N. and Davis, G. C. 1992. Posttraumatic stress disorder in an urban population of young adults: Risk factors for chronicity. *American Journal of Psychiatry* 149(5):671–675.

Brown, P. J., Recupero, P. R., and Stout, R. 1995. PTSD substance abuse comorbidity and treatment utilization. *Addictive Behaviours* 20(2):251–254.

Carey, M. P., Carey, K. B., and Meisler, A. W. 1991. Psychiatric symptoms in mentally ill chemical abusers. *The Journal of Nervous and Mental Disease* 179(3):136–138.

Chu, J. A. 1992. The therapeutic roller coaster: Dilemmas in the treatment of childhood abuse survivors. *Journal of Psychotherapy Practice and Research* (1):351–370.

Cornell, W. F. and Olio, K. A. 1991. Integrating affect in treatment with adult survivors of physical and sexual abuse. *American Journal of Orthopsychiatry* 61(1):59–69.

Cottler, L. B., Compton III, W. M., Mager, D., Spitznagel, E. L., and Janca, A. 1992. Posttraumatic stress disorder among substance users from the general population. *American Journal of Psychiatry* 149(5):664–670.

Dansky, B. S., Saladin, M. E., Brady, K. T., Kilpatrick, D. C., and Resnick, H. S. 1995. Prevalence of victimization and posttraumatic stress disorder among women with substance use disorder: A comparison of telephone and in-person assessment samples. *International Journal of the Addictions* 30:1079–1099.

Dunn, G. E., Paolo, A. M., Ryan. J. J., and Van Fleet, J. 1993. Dissociative symptoms in a substance abuse population. *American Journal of Psychiatry* 150(7):1043–1047.

Evans, K. and Sullivan, J. M. *Treating Addicted Survivors of Trauma.* New York: Guilford Press, 1995.

Everett, B. and Gallop, R. *The Link Between Childhood Trauma and Mental Illness: Effective Interventions for Health Professionals.* London: Sage Publications, 2001.

Foa, E. B. and Rothbaum, B. O. *Treating the Trauma of Rape: Cognitive-Behavioral Therapy for PTSD.* New York: Guilford Press, 1998.

Fullilove, M., Fullilove, R. E., Smith, M., Winkler, K., Michael, C., Panzer, P. G., and Wallace, R. 1993. Violence, trauma, and posttraumatic stress disorder among women drug users. *Journal of Traumatic Stress* 6(4):533–543.

Grilo, C. M., Martino, S., Walker, M. L., Becker, D. F., Edell, W., and McGlashan, T. H. 1997. Psychiatric comorbidity differences in male and female adult psychiatric inpatients with substance use disorders. *Comprehensive Psychiatry* 38(3):155–159.

Harrison, S. and Carver, V. *Alcohol and Drug Problems: A Practical Guide for Counsellors.* Toronto: Centre for Addiction and Mental Health, 2004.

Haskell, L. *First Stage Trama Treatment: A Guide for Mental Health Professionals Working with Women.* Toronto: Centre for Addiction and Mental Health, 2003.

Herman, L. H. *Trauma and Recovery.* USA: Harper Collins Publications, 1992.

Kaufman, E. 1989. The psychotherapy of dually diagnosed patients. *Journal of Substance Abuse Treatment* 6:9–18.

Kaschak, E. *Engendered lives: A New Psychology of Women's Experience.* New York: Basic Books, 1992.

Laub, D. and Auerhahn, N. C. 1993. Knowing and not knowing massive psychic trauma: Forms of traumatic memory. *International Journal of Psychoanalysis* 74:287–302.

Lyon, E. 1993. Hospital staff reactions to accounts by survivors of childhood abuse. *American Journal of Orthopsychiatry* 63(3):410–416.

McCann, I. L. and Pearlman, L. A. *Psychological Trauma and the Adult Survivor. Theory, Therapy and Transformation.* New York: Brunner/Mazel Publications, 1990.

Miller, A. *The Drama of the Gifted Child: The Search for the True Self.* New York: Basic Books, 1994.

Miller, A. *The Untouched Key: Tracing Childhood Trauma in Creativity and Destructiveness.* New York: Anchor Books, Doubleday, 1990.

Miller, D. and Guidry, L. *Addictions and Trauma Recovery: Healing the Body, Mind, and Spirit.* New York: W. W. Norton and Company, 2001.

Miller, P. H. and Scholnick, E. K. *Toward Feminist Developmental Psychology.* New York: Routledge, 2000.

Morrow, M. and Chappell, M. *Hearing Women's Voices: Mental Health Care for Women. Women's Mental Health Reports.* Vancouver: British Columbia Centre of Excellence for Women's Health, 1999.

Najavits, L. M. *Seeking Safety. A Treatment Manual for PTSD and Substance Abuse.* New York: Guilford Press, 2002.

Pearlman, L. A. and Saakvitne, K. W. *Trauma and the Therapist. Counter Transference and Vicarious Traumatization in Psychotherapy with Incest Survivors.* New York: W. W. Norton and Company, 1995.

Rieker, P. P. and (Hilberman) Carmen, E. 1986. Victim-to-patient process: The disconfirmation and transformation of abuse. *American Journal of Orthopsychiatry* 56(3):360–370.

Ries, R. K., Fiellin, D. A., Miller, S. C., and Saitz, R. *Addiction Medicine.* New York: Lippincott Williams & Wilkins, 2009.

Saladin, M. E., Brady, K. T., Dansky, B. S., and Kilpatrick, D. G. 1995. Understanding comorbidity between PTSD and substance use disorders: Two preliminary investigations. *Addictive Behaviours* 20(5):643–655.

Saxe, G. N., Van der Kolk, B. A., Berkowitz, R., Chinman, G. C., Hall, K., Lieberg, G., and Schwartz, J. 1993. Dissociative disorders in psychiatric in patients. *American Journal of Psychiatry* 150(7):1037–1042.

Substance Abuse and Mental Health Services Administration. *Results from the 2008 National Survey on Drug Use and Health: National Findings.* Rockville, MD: Office of Applied Studies, NSDUH Series H-36, HHS Publication No. SMA 09-4434, 2009.

Triffleman, E. G., Marmar, C. R., Delucchi, K. L., and Ronfeldt, H. 1995. Childhood trauma and posttraumatic stress disorder in substance abuse patients. *The Journal of Nervous and Mental Disease* 183(3):172–176.

Van der Kolf, B. *Psychological Trauma.* Washington, DC: American Psychiatric Publishing, Inc., 1987.

Windle, M., Windle, R. C., Scheidt, D. M., and Miller, G. B. 1995. Physical and sexual abuse and associated mental disorders among alcoholic patients. *American Journal of Psychiatry* 152(9):1322–1328.

Wolfe, J. and Chrestman, K. R. 1996. Characteristics of posttraumatic stress disorder-alcohol abuse comorbidity in women. *Journal of Substance Abuse* 8(3):335–346.

Zweben, J. E., Westley Clark, H., and Smith, D. E. 1994. Traumatic experiences and substance abuse: Mapping the territory. *Journal of Psychoactive Drugs* 26(4):327–344.

Internet Resources
Seeking Safety
www.seekingsafety.org
This site offers information on *Seeking Safety: A Treatment Manual*

for PTSD and Substance Abuse (Najavits 2002) as well as the research projects completed and in progress using this model.

Sidran Institute
www.sidran.org
Sidran Institute is a nonprofit organization that provides information to support people with traumatic stress conditions and to help educate mental health professionals and the public.

PILOTS Database
www.ncptsd.org/publications/pilots/index.html
PILOTS is a bibliographical database covering Published International Literature on Traumatic Stress.

International Society of Traumatic Studies
www.istss.org
The International Society for Traumatic Stress Studies offers fact sheets on traumatic loss and the emotional response both for professionals and for the public.

Yoga Research and Education Centre
www.yrec.org and *www.iayt.org*
Founded in 1996 by Georg Feuerstein, YREC is a nonprofit corporation dedicated to making the authentic teachings of traditional Hindu, Buddhist, and Jaina Yoga accessible to sincere students everywhere.

Chapter Two: My Story

Buddha's Teachings. *The Noble Eigthfold Path.* London: Axiom Publishing, 2005.
Campbell, S. S. *Call to Heal: Traditional Healing Meets Modern Medicine in Southern Africa Today.* California: Zebra Press, 1998.
Farmer, S. D. *Animal Spirit Guides.* New York: Hay House, Inc., 2006.

Fontana, D. *Learn to Meditate*. San Francisco: Chronicle Books, 1999.

Frankl, V. E. *Man's Search for Meaning*. New York:Washington Square Press, 1984.

Helminski, K. *The Knowing Heart: A Sufi Path of Transformation*. Boston: Shambhala, 2000.

Iyengar, B. K. S. *Iyengar the Yoga Master*. Boston and London: Shambhala, 2007.

King, M. L. Jr. *I Have a Dream*. San Francisco: Harper San Francisco, 1992.

Losier, M. J. *Law of Attraction*. New York: Wellness Central, 2007.

Malidoma, P. S.*The Healing Wisdom of Africa.* New York: Penguin Putman, 1999.

Mitchell, S. *Bhagavad Gita*. New York: Harmony Books, 2000.

Moore, T. *Care of the Soul*. New York: Harper Perennial, 1992.

Santorelli, S. *Heal Thy Self*. New York: Random House, 1999.

Sharma, R. *The Monk Who Sold His Ferrari*. Toronto: Harper Collins Publishers, 2007.

Thich Nhat Hanh. *Be Still and Know: Reflections from Living Buddha, Living Christ*. New York: Riverhead Books, 1996.

Van Praagh, J. *Meditations*. New York: Simon and Schuster, 2003.

Villoldo, A. *Courageous Dreaming: How Shamans Dream the World Into Being*. New York: Hay House, 2008.

Villoldo, A. *The Four Insights*. London: Hay House, 2007.

Wilber, K. *A Sociable God*. Boston: Shambhala, 2005.

Williamson, M. *The Gift of Change*. New York: Harper One, 2004.

Yalom, I. D. *The Gift of Therapy.* New York: Perennial Publications, 2003.

Yalom, I. D. *Momma and the Meaning of Life.* New York: Perennial Publications, 2000.

Zukav, G. *Soul to Soul: Communications from the Heart*. New York: Free Press, 2007.

Chapter Three: Addiction and Abuse

Everett, B. and Gallop, R. *The Link Between Childhood Trauma and Mental Illness: Effective Interventions for Health Professionals.* London: Sage Publications, 2001.

Morrow, M. and Chappell, M. *Hearing Women's Voices: Mental Health Care for Women. Women's Mental Health Reports.* Vancouver: British Columbia Centre of Excellence for Women's Health, 1999.

Najavits, L. M. *Seeking Safety: A Treatment Manual for PTSD and Substance Abuse.* New York: Guilford Press, 2002.

Poole, N. and Greaves, L. *Highs and Lows: Canadian Perspective on Women and Substance Use.* Toronto: Centre for Addiction and Mental Health Publishers, 2007.

Ries, R. K., Fiellin, D. A., Miller, S. C., and Saitz, R. *Addiction Medicine* . New York: Lippincott Williams & Wilkins, 2009.

Van der Kolf, B. *Psychological Trauma.* Washington, DC: American Psychiatric Publishing, 1987.

Zimmer, L., and Morgan, J. P. *Marijuana Myths Marijuana Facts.* New York: Lindesmith Center, 1997.

Chapter Four: Mika's Healing

Carroll-Johnson, R. M., Gorman, L. M., and Bush, N. J. *Psychosocial Nursing Care: Along the Cancer Continuum.* Pittsburgh: Oncology Nursing Press, 1998.

Frankl, V. E. *Man's Search for Meaning.* New York: Washington Square Press, 1984.

Iyengar, B. K. S. *Light on Yoga.* London: Thorsons, 2001.

Worden, J. W. *Grief Counseling and Grief Therapy.* New York: Springer Publishing Company, 1991.

Chapter Five: Emma Garth

Everett, B. and Gallop, R. *The Link Between Childhood Trauma and Mental Illness: Effective Interventions for Health Professionals.* London: Sage Publications, 2001.

Engel, B. *The Emotionally Abusive Relationship*. New Jersey: John Wiley & Sons, 2002.

Miller, A. *The Drama of the Gifted Child: The Search for the True Self.* New York: Basic Books, 1994.

Miller, A. *The Untouched Key: Tracing Childhood Trauma in Creativity and Destructiveness*. New York: Doubleday, 1990.

Morrow, M. and Chappell, M. *Hearing Women's Voices: Mental Health Care for Women. Women's Mental Health Reports.* Vancouver: British Columbia Centre of Excellence for Women's Health, 1999.

Van der Kolf, B. *Psychological Trauma.* Washington, DC: American Psychiatric Publishing, 1987.

Chapter Six: Highway to Heaven

Bennett, G. A. and Higgins, D. S. (1999). Accidental overdose among injecting drug users in Dorset, UK. *Addiction* 94(8):1179–1189.

Darke, S. and Hall, W. (2003). Heroin overdose: research and evidence-based intervention. *Journal of Urban Health* 80:189–200.

Everett, B. and Gallop, R. *The Link Between Childhood Trauma and Mental Illness: Effective Interventions for Health Professionals.* London: Sage Publications, 2001.

Kerr, T., Tyndall, M. W., Lai, C., Montaner, J. S. G., and Wood, E. (2006). Drug-related overdoses within a medically supervised safer injection facility. *International Journal of Drug Policy* (595):1–6.

Lowenthal, R. *One-Way Ticket: Our Son's Addiction to Heroin.* New York: Beaufort Books, 2003.

Ries, R. K., Fiellin, D. A., Miller, S. C., and Saitz, R. *Addiction Medicine.* New York: Lippincott Williams & Wilkins, 2009.

Van der Kolf, B. *Psychological Trauma.* Washington, DC: American Psychiatric Publishing, 1987.

Chapter Seven: Concurrent Disorders

Breslau, N. and Davis, G. C. 1992. Posttraumatic stress disorder in an urban population of young adults: Risk factors for chronicity. *American Journal of Psychiatry* 149(5):671–675.

Brown, P. J., Recupero, P. R., and Stout, R. 1995. PTSD Substance abuse comorbidity and treatment utilization. *Addictive Behaviours* 20(2):251–254.

Carey, M. P., Carey, K. B., and Meisler, A. W. 1991. Psychiatric symptoms in mentally ill chemical abusers. *The Journal of Nervous and Mental Disease* 179(3):136–138.

Chu, J. A. 1992. The therapeutic roller coaster: Dilemmas in the treatment of childhood abuse survivors. *Journal of Psychotherapy Practice and Research* (1):351–370.

Cornell, W. F. and Olio, K. A. 1991. Integrating affect in treatment with adult survivors of physical and sexual abuse. *American Journal of Orthopsychiatry* 61(1):59–69.

Cournos F., Empfield, M., Horwath, E., et al. 1991. HIV prevalence among patients admitted to two psychiatric hospitals. *American Journal of Psychiatry* 148:1225–1230.

Cottler, L. B., Compton III, W. M., Mager, D., Spitznagel, E. L., and Janca, A. 1992. Posttraumatic stress disorder among substance users from the general population. *American Journal of Psychiatry* 149(5):664–670.

Dansky, B. S., Saladin, M. E., Brady, K. T., Kilpatrick, D. C., and Resnick, H. S. 1995. Prevalence of victimization and posttraumatic stress disorder among women with substance use disorder: A comparison of telephone and in-person assessment samples. *International Journal of the Addictions* 30:1079–1099.

Dunn, G. E., Paolo, A. M., Ryan. J. J., and Van Fleet, J. 1993. Dissociative symptoms in a substance abuse population. *American Journal of Psychiatry* 150(7):1043–1047.

Evans, K. and Sullivan, J. M. *Treating Addicted Survivors of Trauma.* New York: Guilford Press, 1995.

Everett, B. and Gallop, R. *The Link Between Childhood Trauma and*

Mental Illness: Effective Interventions for Health Professionals.
London: Sage Publications, 2001.

Harrison, S. and Carver, V. *Alcohol and Drug Problems: A Practical
Guide for Counsellors.* Toronto: Centre for Addiction and Mental
Health, 2004.

Haskell, L. *First Stage Trauma Treatment: A Guide for Mental Health
Professionals Working with Women.* Toronto: Centre for Addiction
and Mental Health, 2003.

Herman, L. H. *Trauma and Recovery.* New York: Harper Collins
Publications, 1992.

Kaufman, E. 1989. The psychotherapy of dually diagnosed patients.
Journal of Substance Abuse Treatment 6:9–18.

Kofoed, L.L., Kania, J., Walsh, T., et al. 1986. Outpatient treatment
of patients with substance abuse and coexisting psychiatric
disorders. *American Journal of Psychiatry* 143:867–872.

Laub, D. and Auerhahn, N. C. 1993. Knowing and not knowing massive
psychic trauma: Forms of traumatic memory. *International
Journal of Psychoanalysis* 74:287–302.

Miller, A. *The Drama of the Gifted Child: The Search for the True Self.*
New York: Basic Books, 1994.

Miller, A. *The Untouched Key: Tracing Childhood Trauma in Creativity
and Destructiveness.* New York: Doubleday, 1990.

Miller, D. and Guidry, L. *Addictions and Trauma Recovery: Healing
the Body, Mind, and Spirit.* New York: W. W. Norton & Company,
2001.

Najavits, L. M. *Seeking Safety. A Treatment Manual for PTSD and
Substance Abuse.* New York:Guilford Press, 2002.

Ries, R. K., Fiellin, D. A., Miller, S. C., and Saitz, R. *Addiction Medicine
.* New York: Lippincott Williams & Wilkins, 2009.

Saladin, M. E., Brady, K. T., Dansky, B. S., and Kilpatrick, D. G. 1995.
Understanding comorbidity between PTSD and substance use
disorders: Two preliminary investigations. *Addictive Behaviours.*
20(5):643–655.

Triffleman, E. G., Marmar, C. R., Delucchi, K. L., and Ronfeldt, H.
1995. Childhood trauma and posttraumatic stress disorder in

substance abuse patients. *The Journal of Nervous and Mental Disease* 183(3):172–176.

Van der Kolf, B. *Psychological Trauma.* Washington, DC: American Psychiatric Publishing, 1987.

Chapter Eight: Violence in Marginalized Communities

Asante, M. K. *The Afrocentric Idea.* Philadelphia: Temple University Press, 1998.

Brown, E. *A Taste of Power.* New York: Doubleday, 1992.

King, M. L. Jr. *I Have a Dream.* San Francisco: Harper San Francisco, 1992.

Tonry, M. and Moore, M. H. *Youth Violence.* Chicago: University of Chicago Press, 1998.

Shamsie, J., Nicholl, S., and Madsen, K. C. *Antisocial and Violent Youth.* Canada: Lugus Publications, 1999.

Wagner, E. F. and Waldron, H. B. *Innovations in Adolescent Substance Abuse Interventions.* Amsterdam: Pergamon, 2001.

Winks, R. W. *The Blacks in Canada a History.* Montréal: McGill-Queen's University Press, 1997.

Chapter Nine: Altered Body Image

Andy, C., Flake, D., French, L. 2005. Clinical inquiries: Do insulin-sensitizing drugs increase ovulation rates for women with PCOS? *Journal of Family Practice* 156:159–60.

BBC News World Edition. 2003. The diet business.

Cope, S. *Yoga and the Quest for the True Self.* New York: Bantam Books, 1999.

Desikachar, T. K. V. *The Heart of Yoga.* Rochester, VT: Inner Traditions International, 1999.

Freke, T. *Spiritual Traditions.* New York: Sterling Publishers , 2000.

Iyengar, B. K. S. *Light on Yoga.* New York: Schocken Books, 1979.

Iyengar, B. K. S. *Yoga: The Path to Holistic Health.* London: Dorling Kindersley Limited, 2001.

Schiffmann, E. *Yoga: The Spirit and Practice of Moving into Stillness.* New York: Pocket Books, 1996.

Scott, J. *Ashtanga Yoga*. New York: Three Rivers Press, 2000.

Tan, S., Hahn, S., Benson, S., et al. 2007. Metformin improves polycystic ovary syndrome irrespective of pre-treatment insulin resistance. *European Journal of Endocrinology* 157(5):669–76.

Chapter Ten: Healing Is Revealing

Frankl, V. E. *Man's Search for Meaning*. New York: Washington Square Press, 1984.

Iyengar, B. K. S. *Light on Yoga*. London: Thorsons, 2001.

Losier, M. J. *Law of Attraction*. New York: Wellness Central, 2007.

Miller, A. *The Drama of the Gifted Child: The Search for the True Self*. New York: Basic Books, 1994.

Miller, A. *The Untouched Key: Tracing Childhood Trauma in Creativity and Destructiveness*. New York: Doubleday, 1990.

Santorelli, S. *Heal Thy Self*. New York: Random House, 1999.

Van der Kolf, B. *Psychological Trauma*. Washington, DC: American Psychiatric Publishing, 1987.

Chapter Eleven: Life-Threatening Illness

Barry, D. B. *Psychosocial Nursing Care of Physically Ill Patients and Their Families*. New York: Lippincott, 1996.

Blitzer, A. et al. *Communicating with Cancer Patients and Their Families*. Philadelphia: Charles Press, 1990.

Carroll-Johnson, R. M., Gorman, L. M., and Bush, N. J. *Psychosocial Nursing Care; Along the Cancer Continuum*. Pittsburgh: Oncology Nursing Press, 1998.

Frankl, V. E. *Man's Search for Meaning*. New York: Washington Square Press, 1984.

Kemp, C. *Terminal Illness*. Philadelphia: J.B. Lippincott, 1995.

Otto, S. *Oncology Nursing*. Boston: Mosby, 1991.

Santorelli, S. *Heal Thy Self*. New York: Random House, 1999.

Worden, J. W. *Grief Counseling and Grief Therapy*. New York: Springer Publishing Company, 1991.

Chapter Twelve: Is This Abuse?

Everett, B. and Gallop, R. *The Link Between Childhood Trauma and Mental Illness: Effective Interventions for Health Professionals.* London: Sage Publications, 2001.

Poole, N. and Greaves, L. *Highs and Lows: Canadian Perspective on Women and Substance Use.* Toronto: Centre for Addiction and Mental Health Publishers, 2007.

Ries, R. K., Fiellin, D. A., Miller, S. C., and Saitz, R. *Addiction Medicine.* New York: Lippincott Williams & Wilkins, 2009.

Van der Kolf, B. *Psychological Trauma.* Washington, DC: American Psychiatric Publishing, 1987.

Zimmer, L. and Morgan, J.P. *Marijuana Myths Marijuana Facts.* New York: Lindesmith Center, 1997.

Chapter Thirteen: Group Therapy for Trauma and Addiction

Breslau, N. and Davis, G. C. 1992. Posttraumatic stress disorder in an urban population of young adults: Risk factors for chronicity. *American Journal of Psychiatry.* 149(5):671–675.

Brown, P. J., Recupero, P. R., and Stout, R. 1995. PTSD substance abuse comorbidity and treatment utilization. *Addictive Behaviours.* 20(2):251–254.

Carey, M. P., Carey, K. B., and Meisler, A. W. 1991. Psychiatric symptoms in mentally ill chemical abusers. *The Journal of Nervous and Mental Disease.* 179(3):136–138.

Corey, M. S. and Corey, G. *Groups Process and Practice.* Boston: Brooks/Cole Publishing Company, 1997.

Corey, G. *Case Approach to Counseling and Psychotherapy.* New York: Brooks/Cole Publishing Company, 1996.

Chu, J. A. 1992. The therapeutic roller coaster: Dilemmas in the treatment of childhood abuse survivors. *Journal of Psychotherapy Practice and Research* (1):351–370.

Cornell, W. F. and Olio, K. A. 1991. Integrating affect in treatment with adult survivors of physical and sexual Abuse. *American Journal of Orthopsychiatry* 61(1): 59–69.

Cournos, F., Empfield, M., Horwath, E., et al. 1991. HIV prevalence among patients admitted to two psychiatric hospitals. *American Journal of Psychiatry* 148:1225–1230.

Cottler, L. B., Compton III, W. M., Mager, D., Spitznagel, E. L., and Janca, A. 1992. Posttraumatic stress disorder among substance users from the general population. *American Journal of Psychiatry.* 149(5):664–670.

Dansky, B. S., Saladin, M. E., Brady, K. T., Kilpatrick, D. C., and Resnick, H. S. 1995. Prevalence of victimization and posttraumatic stress disorder among women with substance use disorder: A comparison of telephone and in-person assessment samples. *International Journal of the Addictions* 30:1079–1099.

Dunn, G. E., Paolo, A. M., Ryan, J. J., and Van Fleet, J. 1993. Dissociative symptoms in a substance abuse population. *American Journal of Psychiatry* 150(7):1043–1047.

Evans, K. and Sullivan, J. M. *Treating Addicted Survivors of Trauma.* New York: Guilford Press, 1995.

Everett, B. and Gallop, R. *The Link Between Childhood Trauma and Mental Illness: Effective Interventions for Health Professionals.* London: Sage Publications, 2001.

Harrison, S. and Carver, V. *Alcohol and Drug Problems: A Practical Guide for Counsellors.* Toronto: Centre for Addiction and Mental Health, 2004

Haskell, L. *First Stage Trauma Treatment: A Guide for Mental Health Professionals Working with Women.* Centre for Addiction and Mental Health, 2003.

Herman, L. H. *Trauma and Recovery.* New York: Harper Collins Publications, 1992.

Kaufman, E. 1989). The psychotherapy of dually diagnosed patients. *Journal of Substance Abuse Treatment* 6:9–18.

Kofoed, L.L., Kania, J., Walsh, T., et al. 1986. Outpatient Treatment of patients with substance abuse and coexisting psychiatric disorders. *American Journal of Psychiatry* 143:867–872.

Laub, D. and Auerhahn, N. C. 1993. Knowing and not knowing massive psychic trauma: Forms of traumatic memory. *International Journal of Psychoanalysis* 74:287–302.

Miller, A. *The Drama of the Gifted Child: The Search for the True Self.* New York: Basic Books, 1994.

Miller, A. *The Untouched Key: Tracing Childhood Trauma in Creativity and Destructiveness.* New York: Doubleday, 1990.

Miller, D. and Guidry, L. *Addictions and Trauma Recovery: Healing the Body, Mind, & Spirit.* New York: W. W. Norton & Company, 2001.

Najavits, L. M. *Seeking Safety. A Treatment Manual for PTSD and Substance Abuse.* New York: Guilford Press, 2002.

Ries, R. K., Fiellin, D. A., Miller, S. C., and Saitz, R. *Addiction Medicine.* New York: Lippincott Williams & Wilkins, 2009.

Saladin, M. E., Brady, K. T., Dansky, B. S., and Kilpatrick, D. G. 1995. Understanding comorbidity between PTSD and substance use disorders: Two preliminary investigations. *Addictive Behaviours* 20(5):643–655.

Triffleman, E. G., Marmar, C. R., Delucchi, K. L., and Ronfeldt, H. 1995. Childhood trauma and posttraumatic stress disorder in substance abuse patients. *The Journal of Nervous and Mental Disease* 183(3):172–176.

Van der Kolf, B. *Psychological Trauma.* Washington, DC: American Psychiatric Publishing, 1987.

Yalom, I. D. *The Theory and Practice of Group Psychotherapy.* New York: Basic Books, 1985.

Zweben, J. E., Westley Clark, H., and Smith, D. E. 1994. Traumatic experiences and substance abuse: Mapping the territory. *Journal of Psychoactive Drugs* 26(4):327–344.

Chapter Fourteen: Death of a Group Member

Bonnie, J. B. 1995. Etiology and management of anger in groups: A psychodynamic view. *International Journal of Group Psychotherapy* 45:275–284.

Collins, G. B. 1993. Contemporary issues in the treatment of alcohol dependence. *Psychiatric Clinics of North America* 16:33–48.

Corey, M. S and Corey, G. *Groups Process and Practice* Boston: Brooks/Cole Publishing Company, 1997.

Corey, G. *Case Approach to Counseling and Psychotherapy.* New York: Brooks/Cole Publishing Company, 1996.

Diagnostic and Statistical Manual Of Mental Disorders, 4th ed. Washington, DC: American Psychiatric Press, 1994.

Flores, P. J. and Mahon, L. 1993. The treatment of addictions in group psychotherapy. *International Journal of Group Psychotherapy* 43:143–156.

Hesselbrock, M. N., Meyer, R. E., and Keener, J. J. 1985. Psychopathology of hospitalized alcoholics. *Archives of General Psychiatry* 42:322–327.

Khantzian, E. J., Halliday, K. S., McAuliffe, W. E. *Addiction and the Vulnerable Self.* New York: Guilford Press, 1990.

Kemker, S. S., Kibel, H. D., and Mahler, J. C. 1993. On becoming oriented to inpatient addiction treatment: Inducing new patient and professionals to the recovery movement. *International Journal of Group Psychotherapy* 43: 285–301.

Kirman, J. H. 1995. Working with anger in groups: A modern analytic approach. *International Journal of Group Psychotherapy* 45:303–329.

Miller, N. S. *Addiction Psychiatry: Current Diagnosis and Treatment.* New York: Wiley-Liss, 1995.

Ries, R. K., Fiellin, D. A., Miller, S. C. and Saitz, R. *Addiction Medicine.* New York: Lippincott Williams & Wilkins, 2009.

Room, R. *Co-occurring Mental Disorders and Addictions: Scientific Evidence on Epidemiology and Treatment Outcomes. Implications for Services in Ontario.* Toronto: Addiction Research Foundation, 1997.

Yalom, I. D. *The Theory and Practice of Group Psychotherapy.* New York: Basic Books, 1985.